HERE'S WHAT TI
ABOUT TI.

"This book could be the *text for the course, HOME CARE 101.* It is exactly what the title implies: a book of basic instruction for any individual who will be providing someone's personal care needs in a natural environment. I would be interested in using it as an *orientation manual* for newly hired CHHAs."

Georgia Simmons, RN, Home Care Coordinator
King's Daughters' Hospital, Home Health and Hospice Services,
Madison, IN

"*Exquisite work.* The author provides a handbook to guide you through each step in the care of the homebound patient. Finally, we have something more than a note from the physician or nurse. *A handbook worth reading and using.*"

Mark E. Abell, BS, PA-C
Author of numerous medical articles and publications,
Ashburn, GA

"An easy-to-read, *invaluable guide* for anyone caring for a loved one at home. As nurse-owners of a home health agency, we plan to '*prescribe' this book* for all of our clients' families!"

Norma Bedford Christie, RN, BNSc
Robin Minor Anderson, RN, BSN, PHN
Baker, Anderson, Christie, Inc, San Franciso, CA

- continue -

"Many books exist that give families general ideas of how to care for a person at home. But when you *really need the details, The Step-by-Step Guide to Caring for the Homebound* will give you what you want. If you can't get a nurse to spend hours teaching you the *nitty gritty of caregiving*, this book is the next best thing."

Sharon Emerson, RN, Administrator
Island Home Nursing, Langley, WA

"You have a great concept in this *easy-to-use* primer for home care. The *figures* and *diagrams* which illustrate the written instructions are *extremely helpful*. The cute comments throughout provide relief from the occasional tedium of care."

Penny Sanchez, RN, BSN, MA, Instructor
Indiana Vocational Technical College. Madison, IN

"Gerrie Hallas' book is an *easy to read, practical,* respectful guide to caring for the homebound patient. The step-by-step instructions are *easy to follow* and *appropriate humor* adds to their effectiveness. The book can be placed nearby for *reference* while accomplishing each task, and *crisp illustrations* further enhance understanding. This book will encourage the typical caregiver to remember that *caring for his or her loved one at home is both possible and rewarding.*"

Paula Limato, BS, Director of Volunteer Services
King's Daughters' Hospital, Home Health & Hospice Services, Madison, IN

THE
STEP–BY–STEP GUIDE
TO
Caring For The
HOMEBOUND

98   99   00   01   8   7   6   6   5   4   3   2

ATTENTION RETAILERS AND CORPORATIONS

This book, and other products supplied by the Publisher, are available at quantity discounts with bulk purchases for education-al use, business or sales promotion, or fund raising. Special books or book excerpts can also be created to fit specific needs. Contact the Publisher for details.

Library of Congress Cataloging-in-Publication Data

Hallas, Gerrie L., 1963-
        The step-by-step guide to caring for the homebound / by
Gerrie L. Hallas ; illustrations by Teresa Herman.
            p.   cm.
        Includes index.
        ISBN 0-944214-12-6 (alk. paper)
        1. Home nursing   I Title
    RT61.H33   1999
    649.8—dc21   98-46054
                                                      CIP

ISBN: 0-944214-12-6

PRINTED IN THE UNITED STATES OF AMERICA

THE
STEP-BY-STEP GUIDE
TO
CARING FOR THE HOMEBOUND

GERRIE L. HALLAS, CMA, MHT, CHHA

ILLUSTRATIONS BY TERESA HERMAN

Published by

ABELexpress
P.O. Box 668
Carnegie, PA 15106

412-279-0672 – 412-279-5012 FAX – 800-542-9001 U.S.A.
ken@abelexpress.com

COVER by
Archer-Ellison Design

800-449-4095
design@bookcovers.com
www.bookcovers.com

ILLUSTRATIONS by
Teresa Herman

412-928-0279

PRINTING & BINDING by
Northeastern Press

800-248-9484
570-488-6272 FAX

This book is dedicated to John's Mamaw and Papaw

CONTENTS

FOREWORD

Changes in the health care delivery system within the United States will soon affect everyone. Government edicts which demand that the medical community deliver "optimal" care to all Americans will trickle down to the individual, who may be left to fend for him or herself.

Since the advent of modern medicine, the delivery of primary healthcare, and of supportive care, had been left in the hands of trained practitioners. Today, under "managed care," hospital and nursing home stays are shorter, and treatment programs - to be completed within specified time limits - demand *optimal* rather than *maximal* care, often regardless of individual needs. Thus, in many cases, patients are released from institutions while still unable to take care of themselves. *(I have seen many a patient discharged from a hospital with only a note from the physician telling the patient what to eat, how to deal with their illness as it progresses, and when to return for a follow-up appointment. No information on how to survive between release date and follow-up date, included!)*

My experiences, mainly in rehabilitation, have given insight into the needs of the patients as they return to their own domicile; while they are usually glad to be home, they are often anxious. Some of the simplest of tasks, which were once second nature or innate to them, are now more difficult, or even tedious.

The list of "Activities of Daily Living," or ADLs - such as combing hair, brushing teeth, making a bed, or washing the body - is extensive. Completion of the list by a patient who has, for example, suffered a stroke or massive heart attack, may be virtually impossible. Thus, the former patient needs assistance. In earlier days, that assistance would be rendered by a home care professional. But the same forces that reduce treatment times and hospital stays also reduce the monies available for professional home care assistance. So, what do you do to care of your loved one, in the absence of professional help? Probably the best thing to do is to acquire a copy of Gerrie Hallas' book, *The Step-by-Step Guide to Caring for the Homebound.*

This book, by a veteran home care professional and trainer, changes everything. For the first time, someone whose illness or disability prevents them from taking care of themselves, has a resource which allows their loved ones to take care of them, in the absence of professional help. The author has taken great pains to explain, in detail, and with numerous illustrations, how untrained persons can perform at home, routines which have heretofore been left to nurses or aides.

Gerrie Hallas' book allows a successful transition from an institution to home and provides straightforward, easy-to-understand directions for delivering care to a homebound individual. Explanations are provided to enhance understanding, and questions are posed to help the reader recognize the importance of certain elements of care.

I am quite sure that you will enjoy the book and that, having read it, you will be well armed to assist the patient who has been left in your hands.

Mark E. Abell, PA-C

ACKNOWLEDGEMENTS

Many, many thanks to those who made this book possible, especially Jennie Dunn, Sheilah Adams, and Kathy Scroggins. Thanks to the nursing department at Southeastern Louisiana University for reviewing this book, as well as to others who took time from their hectic schedules to help make the book the best it could be.

Additional thanks to Dr. DOS, who repeatedly rescued me from the clutches of that infernal machine, my computer. Or rescued it from me!

And of course, my very special thanks to my husband, Mike, for his quiet, constant support in all I do. Thanks for going that last 50 yards.

Gerrie Hallas, author

Thanks to Teresa Herman for converting the author's original drawings and diagrams into detailed, professional illustrations, making it easier for readers to understand the step-by-step instructions.

Thanks to Jessica Abel for her many hours in helping to edit this book and in fine tuning the layout.

Ken Abel, ABELexpress, publisher

INTRODUCTION

Health care costs are rising.

Cost-conscious, managed care "gatekeepers" are telling hospitals to send patients home sooner.

A home health nurse may come once or twice a week for a few months or a few weeks. Or maybe not at all.

Perhaps you put the patient in a nursing home. But the money runs out and they have to return to *your* home.

And maybe . . . there isn't any insurance at all.

Let's face it. You're on your own.

You know they have to be bathed and fed . . . and exercised. And maybe they have medical needs that need to be tended to.

But *how* do you do these things? What *else* must you do? What *shouldn't* you do? If you hire someone, how do you know if *they* know what to do?

The answers to these questions - the hows, the whys and why nots, the do's and don'ts - are what this book is all about.

CHAPTER 1

THE PRELIMINARIES

Referring to the Patient

To simplify matters, I will refer to the patient as *Alice* throughout this book.

Except for certain obvious differences, care for men and women is the same. There have been men named Alice ... I've just never had the pleasure of meeting any of them.

About The Caregiver

An essential quality in a caregiver is patience. It may be easier and faster for *you* to do everything for your patient; but having the patience to stand back as she tries to do it herself has the reward of boosting both her emotional and physical strength.

Before We Go Any Further, Let's Talk About *Gloves*

Be it friend, family member, or someone you are hired to care for, wear rubber gloves during personal care.

Why?

Because bacteria, which *WILL* be on your hands, can cause harm to Alice. And because bacteria which *WILL* be on, or in, Alice, can cause harm to you. In fact, not only can some of these bacteria cause infection in cuts and scrapes, but certain bacteria in human feces can cause serious illness, even death!

Remember:

- Gloves protect your hands (and the rest of you) from Alice's germs.

- Gloves protect Alice from germs carried on your hands.

That brings us to hand washing . . . *Do it a lot!*

- Before you prepare Alice's food.

- After you take her plate.

- **Before and after you brush her teeth.**

- **Before and after personal care, *particularly* bathroom visits.**

That's a lot of hand washing. And it will tend to dry your skin, so use a *moisturizing* antibacterial soap. Don't feel compelled to use a name brand - generics usually have the same active ingredients.

Following the Step-by-Step Instructions

In most situations where we offer step-by-step instructions, we will number the instructions sequentially solely to make it easier to find your place once you look away from the book. *("OK, we were about to start number 5 before the deliveryman came to the door.")*

WRITE NOTES HERE

CHAPTER 2

PERSONAL CARE & BATHING

Let's start with one of the most basic procedures in caring for a homebound patient: bathing and providing personal care. Tips are included to make these procedures easier and less embarrassing for both patient and caregiver. *Note that although you want the patient to remain as independent as possible, assisting her with bathing conserves her strength for other activities.*

Your first step before bathing or transferring Alice is to take off your - *and her* - watches and jewelry. Watch buckles, rings with protruding settings, and pins, can scratch you or Alice.

Keep your nails fairly short to reduce the likelihood of scratching her. And keep Alice's nails trimmed to prevent your being scratched.

Also remember to practice good body mechanics - basically, this means *good posture* - during all aspects of patient care. In particular, work at a comfortable height so you don't have to stoop or slouch to reach Alice as you bathe her. And use the strength of your legs, not your back, when you transfer Alice. You should perform these movements with your feet roughly shoulder width apart, to provide a broad base of support. Avoid reaching or stretching as these also inflict strain on back muscles.

Specific suggestions for good body mechanics during transfers are offered in *Chapter 15: Getting Out of Bed.*

The Bed Bath

PREPARATION

Supplies needed:

- 2 wash cloths, soap, lotion, powder, deodorant, etc.
- 3 towels (2 large, 1 medium)
- Pan or basin of warm water - to be changed as needed

Arrange your supplies in a convenient location - on a chair or card table, bed table or chest. Make sure the room is warm and free from drafts.

Be sure Alice has privacy for her bath. She may be in a hospital bed which ended up in the living room due to lack of space in the bedroom, so be sure to close blinds or curtains. If there are others in the house, be sure they know it is bath time so they may occupy themselves elsewhere.

Gather the clothes Alice will be putting on after her bath and have them nearby, yet out of the drip zone. Alice can dress as you go. This keeps her from getting chilled and eliminates a lot of extra rolling around. Dressing as you go is especially important for patients who suffer extreme fatigue or severe pain, as is frequently the case with the terminally ill.

If Alice is in a hospital bed, you can make it easier for Alice – and for you – by raising the head. Or elevating the entire bed. To prevent back strain for you, perhaps Alice can sit up on the bed, or swing over to the side.

Undress or uncover only what is being washed. Keep the rest dressed or covered with a large towel.

As you wash, look for reddened, blistered or broken areas in the skin. Commonly known as bed sores, these should be treated promptly by a medical professional, be it Alice's doctor or home health nurse. *Contrary to formerly taught treatment methods, massage of reddened areas is <u>not recommended</u>.* Massage creates shearing or friction, which actually causes injury.

These reddened, blistered or broken areas, known as *pressure sores,* or in medical terms, *decubitis ulcers,* are usually caused by pressure, hence the name. But they can also be caused by the friction that results from rubbing against braces, casts, catheter, oxygen tubing, or other devices . . . or even clothing and sheets. Information on where to look for pressure sores, how to prevent them and what to do if Alice develops them is covered in much greater detail in *Chapter 13: Decubitis Ulcers: Prevention & Treatment.*

HOW TO DO IT – STEP-BY-STEP

HEAD & UPPER BODY

1. Start with Alice's face and neck. Encourage her to perform as much of the bath as possible herself. Use one washcloth for soaping, the other for rinsing. Wash thoroughly yet gently. Rinse and dry with the medium size towel - it is easier to handle than the larger ones.

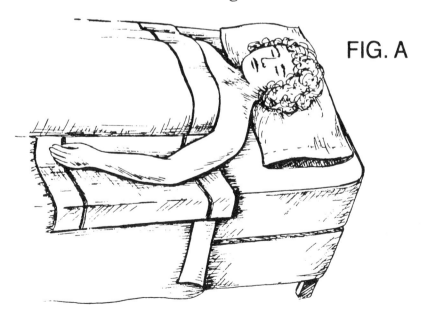

FIG. A

2. Proceed to hands, arms and underarms. Spread a large towel under the parts being washed to keep the bed dry. $\boxed{See\ Figure\ A}$ Repeat as described in (1) above.

3. Use powder, corn starch, deodorant and perfume on already washed and dried areas to suit Alice's tastes; *but note that powder and perfumes may not be suitable if she has respiratory complications.*

   Powder can be especially irritating - don't sprinkle it on; instead, apply with a powder puff or your hand, so there is less drift. To prevent the unpleasant shock of cold lotion, warm the bottle in the basin of water or rub it between your hands before applying.

4. This is a good time to shave Alice's underarms, because hairs are softened by bathing. Refer to *Chapter 5: Shaving.* Use soap or shaving foam/gel. Rinse well and dry. Apply powder or deodorant. Remember to apply powder with a powder puff, or sprinkle it into your hand; don't sprinkle it on Alice.

5. Change the water.

6. Wash and rinse chest and stomach. Use extra care on the navel and under breasts, behind ears and in skin folds. These areas trap perspiration and can easily become irritated. If neglected, the skin breaks down making it vulnerable to infection and bleeding. As you bathe Alice,

look for red, irritated areas behind ears, under breasts and in skin folds. For men, pay special attention to any skin folds on the penis and around the scrotum, which also trap urine and perspiration. See *Chapter 3: Peri Care: Special Care for the Genital Area,* for more information.

7. Dry gently. Blot, rather than rub, sensitive areas. Apply lotion, powder and deodorant as desired by patient. Avoid lotion in skin folds unless they are dry and scaly. Cover with large towel to prevent chill.

8. If Alice is unable to sit up, help her to roll on her side. *(See Chapter 11: Urinary Incontinence, Using a Draw Sheet to Turn Alice, for ways to assist turning.).*

9. Tuck a large towel under her back to keep bedding dry. See *Figure B* The towel can be flipped up over her back to prevent chilling while rinsing wash cloths or performing other types of care. Wash, rinse and dry.

FIG. B

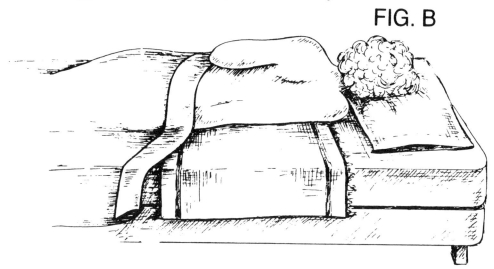

10. Spend a few minutes giving a back rub with lotion, followed by a light dusting with powder. Remember to powder puff, not sprinkle! The powder is refreshing and allows clothing to slip on more easily. If there are no signs of skin breakdown *(reddened skin, blisters or broken skin)* gently massage to improve circulation.

LOWER BODY & EXTREMITIES

1. Dress Alice's top half but don't pull dresses/gowns down over hips yet. Cover hips with one of the large towels. Let Alice rest for a few moments while you get a fresh basin of water.

2. Time for Alice to lie on her back. Now let's see some leg, just one at a time. Pull down and remove pajama bottoms or push them up over knees and thighs. Gowns can be pushed up - drape a towel over Alice's lap, if need be. Spread a large towel under the leg being washed to protect bedding.

3. Wash, rinse, and dry each leg and foot. Take care when putting Alice's foot into, and removing it from, the basin. Remember to spread a large towel under both the basin and Alice's leg to catch the drips – which could be dangerously slippery for both you *and* Alice. You may be able to just rest the basin on the bed and place Alice's foot in it by bending her leg at the knee. A rectangular, flat bottom basis is best if you are placing it on the bed. A waterproof

(rubberized) mat underneath the towel, which is under the basin, will help keep the bedding dry if there are major splashes or the basin tips over.

4. Inspect Alice's feet and legs for signs of decubitus, especially on the inner sides of Alice's knees, heels and ankles. If there are no reddened areas, massage with lotion.

5. To prevent pressure sores from occurring, place a small pillow or folded towel between Alice's knees or ankles when she lies on her side. While inspecting Alice's feet, also look for scrapes, torn or ingrown nails, and crud (hey, we don't have to use a medical term for *everything!*) between toes.

6. If Alice can sit on the side of the bed, put the basin on the floor. Soak her feet while you bathe her legs. Squeeze lots of water over her legs with the washcloth or use a small cup to dip and pour. After Alice removes her feet from the basin, *set the basin out of the way* (or would you really enjoy cleaning up a gallon of water from the floor!?!) and dry her feet thoroughly. Use a small towel or a dry washcloth to dry between the toes - no tickling allowed.

7. Use lotion and powder to individual tastes. Don't get a lot of lotion between her toes - it can lead to fungal infections, particularly in hot, humid weather.

MIDSECTION

1. Now it's time to remove Alice's pajama bottoms or underwear. If Alice is bed bound, she lies on her back, knees bent and feet flat on the bed. If possible, Alice raises her hips while you slip the clothing down. Be sure to slide a large towel under her hips to keep the bed dry. *See Figure C* A hand supporting her lower back or gently pushing down on her knees can provide an extra boost. Next, Alice lowers her hips and straightens her legs (one at a time, to prevent back strain) to finish removing the garment. *This can all be accomplished under the privacy of the sheet or a large towel.*

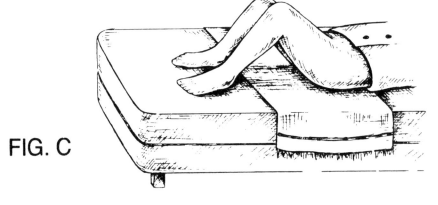

FIG. C

If Alice can't raise her hips, turn her to one side and slip that side of the clothing (pajama bottoms, panties, etc.) down as far as it will go. Turn her to her other side and repeat the process. It may take a couple of turns back and forth. While making these turns, place a towel under her hips to keep the bedclothes dry. Do this by rolling the towel halfway up from one end. While Alice is turned on her side, put the rolled side against her. *See Figure D1*

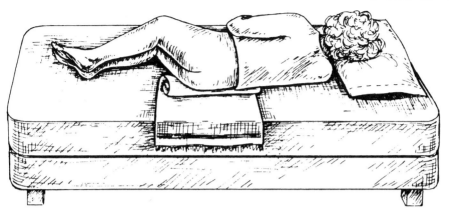

FIG. D-1

2. Roll her to her other side, over the rolled towel. Then unroll the towel. *See Figure D2*

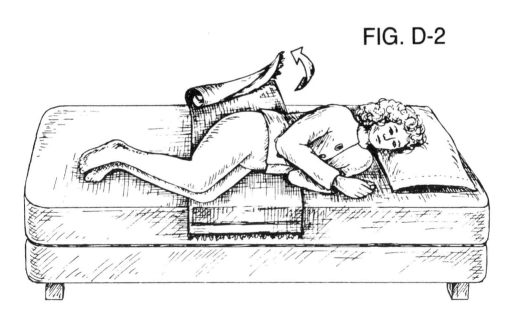

FIG. D-2

3. Turn Alice onto her back again. Make sure she's covered. Change the water. Alice probably needs a brief rest following all of that turning anyway.

4. **Wash and rinse genital area well, keeping Alice covered as much as possible. For both men and women, always wash front to back. This means washing the genital area before the anal area. This is especially important in women, for whom this precaution may prevent vaginal infections or urinary tract infections (UTI's).**

5. **Dry thoroughly. Avoid use of lotion and keep powder to a minimum in this area because it may also contribute to urinary tract and/or vaginal infections. Use powder or cornstarch primarily in creases of thighs to absorb moisture and prevent chafing.** *See Figure E* **Special care for men will be discussed in** *Chapter 3: Peri Care: Special Care for the Genital Area.*

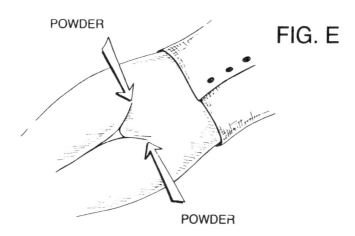

POWDER

FIG. E

POWDER

6. **Turn Alice on her side. Wash hips, then buttocks and anal area.** *Note: washcloths may seem soft to you, but when rubbed over anal area they may feel like sandpaper to Alice; be gentle in sensitive areas! If necessary, substitute baby wipes for a softer touch.*

7. Rinse and dry thoroughly. Lotion will soothe. Keep it out of folds and creases - too much moisture can cause irritation. Powder will help clothing slide on easier.

8. Help Alice slip on clean underwear. Gowns/dresses can be pulled down or pants pulled up. Again, it may take some rolling from side to side to get Alice's clothing on straight.

Shower Chairs (Benches)

If Alice is able to walk fairly well, consider using a shower chair. These chairs are available from medical supply companies and even some department stores. Many home health agencies use them - perhaps you can borrow one for a test drive. Used ones are often discovered in the classified ads and even at yard sales. If you do obtain a used one, be sure it is clean and sturdy.

In my home health agency days, I showered patients seated on everything from 3-legged stools to plastic lawn chairs. To be safe, the seat must be level in the tub or shower. If it tips, don't use it. A simple "rule of thumb": if the stool or bench is something on which Alice couldn't safely sit if it were in her living room, don't use it for her shower.

There are two basic bench types, *regular* and *transfer*. The regular bench fits completely inside the tub. If Alice is able to step over the edge of the tub with/without your support, a regular bath bench should be fine. She just steps into the tub, then sits down on the bench.

The chair illustrated here is a padded transfer bench. Part of it extends outside the tub, making it the safest alternative. This also makes it more expensive and somewhat messy; it's hard not to get any water on the floor. Consider spreading an old towel on the floor next to the tub *after* Alice gets in - so Alice doesn't trip on it. Remove it *before* she exits the tub . . . for the same reason.

To use a transfer bench, Alice sits down on the part of the bench outside of the tub. See Figure F1 She pivots her knees toward the tub, lifting her first foot into the tub. See Figure F2 Next, Alice shifts her hips farther over on the seat, then brings her other foot into the tub. See Figure F3 Speed is not important here – it's safer to move slowly.

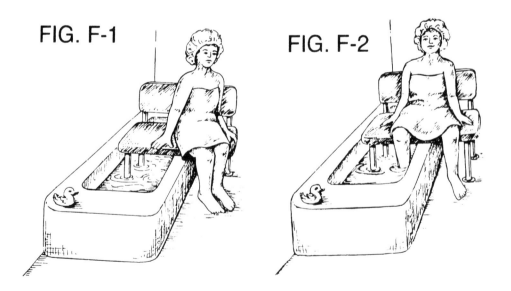

FIG. F-1   FIG. F-2

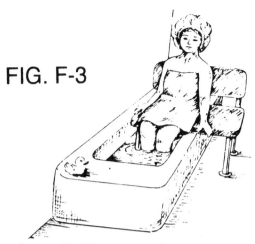

FIG. F-3

If a shower isn't available run a few inches of water in the tub. A large plastic cup or empty margarine tub works very well to dip water, to pour over Alice, as do plastic pitchers with handles. The handle helps you keep a good grip on the pitcher. *(Wet, soapy plastic can become very slippery when you are wearing rubber gloves. You did remember to put them on, didn't you?)*

Another alternative - inexpensive rubber shower hoses are available in many stores. Easily installed, these hoses slip over the faucet. More expensive hand held shower massage units are also available.

To get Alice out of the tub, reverse the procedures described above. First dry her off as much as possible. Alice can wrap up in a robe or towel; *just make sure it won't trip her as she gets out of the tub.* Check the floor for drips and spills. Wipe them up before Alice gets out of the tub so nobody slips and falls.

A safety note. To prevent scalds and burns, always turn the cold water "on" first, and "off" last. Turn the taps on slowly. Then, turn the shower on slowly, after the temperature has been adjusted. Try to point the stream away from Alice until the temperature has been adjusted.

Other safety considerations include non-slip rubber mats *beside* the tub and *inside* the tub, on the floor. Get the type with the little suction feet on the back. Rinse them off and hang them up to dry after Alice's bath, or the mildew monster will attack them. Spray occasionally with disinfectant. I toss mine into the washer with a load of towels or rugs, light on the bleach, in very warm water, hang to dry. Just don't hold me responsible if you forget they're made of rubber and put them in the dryer.

Tub Bath

Don't try a tub bath unless Alice is very steady on her feet. Screw-in or bolt-on hand rails are a good idea. *Non-slip mats are less expensive than a broken hip.* Use them <u>in the tub</u> and <u>next to the tub</u>, instead of a regular bath mat. Remember to hang them up to dry after draining the tub or the mildew monster may attack them.

Whether it's a tub bath or shower, begin with Alice's face and work your way down. Alice leans to one side, then the other to wash the groin and anal areas while seated. Be sure to rinse well. A shower hose makes it much easier. As always, Alice should do as much of the washing as possible. You may only need to wash her back, feet and lower legs.

Check to be sure Alice is washing thoroughly. If Alice is male, he is often embarrassed to ask a female caregiver for help washing private areas. He may pretend he can do it himself. The reality that he cannot must be discovered before skin breakdown occurs. Explain to Mr. Alice why this invasion of his privacy is so important. If necessary, get the home health nurse or a physician to speak with him about the importance of skin care in the genital area.

Drain the tub before Alice gets out. Dry her off as much as possible to prevent chilling and slipping. *Reminder: check for spills and drips on the floor. Wipe them up before Alice gets out of the tub.*

Sometimes Alice can't seem to stand up to get out of the tub. See if she can get on her hands and knees. Support her under the arms and help her to stand.

If that doesn't work, do the following.

1. Get Alice into a sitting position.

2. Kick off your shoes and socks so you don't scratch Alice with your shoe - or get your shoes wet (you're also less likely to slip and fall on top of Alice). Roll up your pant legs.

3. **Stand behind Alice, who should be in a seated position.**

4. **Put one foot in the far side of the tub. Leave the other on the floor outside the tub.**

5. **Bend your knees - don't lean over – and wrap your arms around Alice's chest, underneath her arms. Grasp one wrist with your other hand. _See Figure G_**

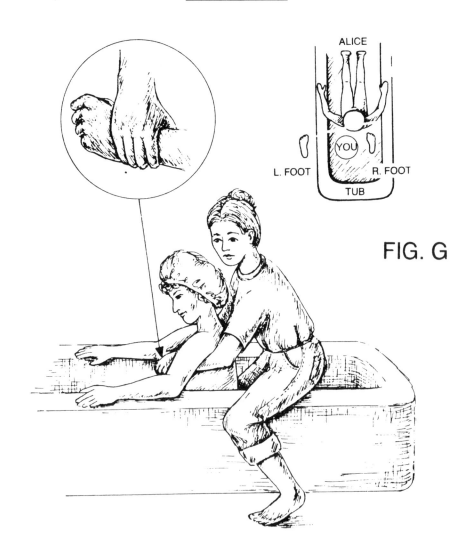

FIG. G

20

6. Straighten your legs, shifting a quarter turn so Alice is sitting on the side of the tub. Keep your feet far apart for good balance.

7. Support Alice while she lifts her feet out, then stands up. You can also lower someone into the tub by reversing this technique. I don't recommend its use on a regular basis.

Don't panic if you can't lift Alice. Dry her off and cover her up with towels or a robe. Make sure she's warm and not injured. Call for help. Alice can slip on a gown or t-shirt or something. If it gets a little wet, so what? It will dry. Better to get <u>help</u> than to get <u>hurt</u>!

WRITE NOTES HERE

CHAPTER 3

PERI CARE: SPECIAL CARE FOR THE GENITAL AREA

For Women

When cleaning up after a visit to the bathroom, always wipe from front to back. This prevents fecal matter from being pushed into the urinary tract or the vagina. This rule should be followed when Alice uses the toilet *(wiping)* and when she bathes *(washing)*.

If Alice is large and her groin area is hard to reach for cleansing, use what hospital aides call a *peri bottle*. It's nothing more than a "squeeze bottle" you fill with warm soapy water which will shoot out in a stream when squeezed. Alice can use this to cleanse her groin, and her vaginal and anal areas, while on the toilet or in the bath. She can also use it while on a bedpan. When finished washing, dump the soapy water, refill with plain water, and rinse well. For a homespun version of the peri bottle, simply recycle a small dishwashing liquid bottle.

For Men - Special Care For The Uncircumcised

What if Alice is an uncircumcised male who is unable to care for himself? It may be embarrassing for Alice or for you. If neglected, painful problems can develop. It is important to learn how to care for him properly.

As with women, wash the genital area before washing the anal area. Carefully pull back the foreskin *(the skin which would be removed during a circumcision)* completely. Gently and thoroughly cleanse with soap and water. Rinse and dry well. A very light layer of petroleum jelly may be applied before the foreskin is pulled back into place. This forms a barrier against moisture. Be careful not to get any into Mr. Alice's *urinary meatus*, doctor technotalk for the urinary opening. Finally, pull the foreskin back into place.

Why put both Alice and yourself through this embarrassment?

1. If not cleansed regularly, the foreskin can trap urine and become very raw, even to the point of bleeding. I've had to salvage a few patients who had reached this state before being admitted to our agency.

2. If not retracted or pulled back regularly, the foreskin can shrink. It slowly strangles Alice's penis. This can also happen if the foreskin is retracted but not returned after washing/urinating. Surgical intervention may be necessary.

3. If the skin is not retracted regularly, it can grow into the skin on the head of Alice's penis. This is called a *skin adhesion.* Besides making good skin care impossible, it creates another problem. It is normal for Mr. Alice to have erections. If the foreskin has adhered to the skin of his penis, Mr. Alice doesn't have enough room to have an erection. This doesn't prevent them from happening. Instead, the urinary opening at the end of Mr. Alice's penis is stretched open when he has an erection. Not only is this painful, it puts him at greater risk of a bladder infection. Surgery may be necessary. Skin adhesions can also occur in uncircumcised or incompletely circumcised infants and children.

WRITE NOTES HERE

CHAPTER 4

SHAMPOOS & HAIR CARE

One of the most important factors in hair care is preparation. Gather your supplies before you start. Make sure the room is warm and free from drafts. Have plenty of towels on hand. In short, *plan ahead.*

In the tub or shower, wash Alice's hair before washing the rest of her body. This is an especially good idea if she uses a conditioner, which tends to build up on the scalp and skin. Rinse well since shampoo and conditioners tend to be very slippery. Of course, if Alice can't get into the bathtub, she can't get her hair washed there either. So . . . .

Shampooing In Bed

Alice can still enjoy a real shampoo even if she is bed bound. Permanents can also be given using the methods we are about to describe.

PREPARATION

A device called a shampoo board is required. There are two types. The example of Figure H1 is inflatable *(rather like a mini-wading pool with a drainage hose).* The example of Figure H2 is a hard plastic board. Both work basically the same way. The hard plastic board is more durable but less comfortable.

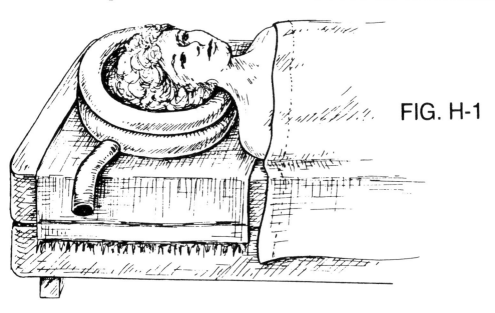

FIG. H-1

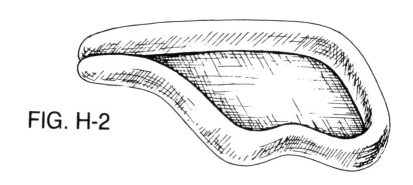

FIG. H-2

Spread a large towel underneath Alice's head and shoulders. Consider putting a large sheet of plastic underneath the towel. A large trash bag split down one side and across the end does the trick nicely. Position the board under Alice's head. You can pad the neck rest of the hard board with a folded wash cloth. Make sure the drain extends past the edge of the bed. *See Figure I* Position a bucket directly underneath the drain. Have one or two basins (or large pitchers) of warm water ready.

FIG. I

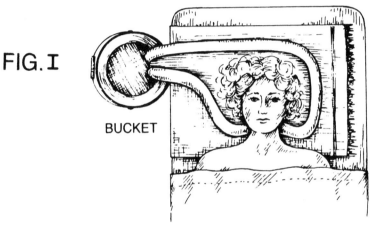

BUCKET

If a shampoo board isn't available, Alice can lie diagonally across the bed, on her back or her stomach, with her head hanging over the edge of the bed. Comfort is the deciding factor between the two positions. First, cover the bed with the plastic and towel. Get everything ready before Alice gets into position. Put a bucket on the floor, beneath her head to catch the water as you pour. This method works best if an extra pair of hands is available to support Alice's head.

HOW TO DO IT – STEP-BY-STEP

1. Using a large plastic cup or pitcher *(plastic so if you bounce the cup in the middle of Alice's forehead you won't knock her cold)* pour enough water over her head to wet hair thoroughly. Pour shampoo into the palm of your hand. Mix in a little water to lather Alice's hair evenly. Work up a good lather.

2. Rinse carefully. Make sure the bucket doesn't overflow. Empty if need be. Rinse well.

3. Lather again or apply conditioner. Blot hair with a towel, then wrap a towel around Alice's hair.

4. Carefully remove the shampoo board - after you went to all that trouble keeping the bed dry, you don't want to mess it up now. *(Wonder how I knew that could happen?)* Let Alice rest a few minutes while you clean up.

Washing Hair at the Sink

If Alice is fairly mobile you can wash her hair at the kitchen sink. If she uses a walker, position it in front of the sink for extra support. *Position a chair directly behind Alice in case she becomes dizzy or tired.*

Check to make sure you have everything you need within easy reach.

1. Turn on the water and adjust the temperature. Alice assumes a stable, supported position, leaning forward with her head turned to one side.

2. Wet her hair with the sprayer or pour water from a large plastic container. A small rolled towel helps prevent drips down Alice's back.

3. After the shampoo Alice can sit in the chair. While she takes a rest or combs her hair, check the floor for drips and puddles. Wipe them up to prevent falls.

Chemical Shampoos

Maybe Alice recently had surgery or is very ill. She doesn't feel up to a regular shampoo. Many drug stores and home health supply retailers offer chemical or dry shampoos which don't need to be rinsed out. Both liquid and spray forms are available.

Follow the product's directions carefully. The liquid form can be very cold . . . so pour some in a cup and warm in the microwave for 15-20 seconds. No microwave? Warm the whole bottle in a bowl of hot water. Test the temperature on your wrist before applying. *(Remember how you used to do that with the baby's bottle?)*

Another alternative is to sprinkle the roots of her hair with baby powder. Work it into scalp with your fingers. Brush thoroughly. The powder absorbs oil and dirt. Don't use powder if Alice has any breathing problems or if Alice won't be able to tolerate a more conventional shampoo soon; over time the powder can accumulate and irritate the scalp, so it must eventually be washed out.

Which of the above is your best bet? Probably the liquid chemical (no rinse) shampoo. The spray version might prove irritating if Alice has respiratory ailments. Baby powder might also be irritating; and it must be washed out sooner or later.

If all else fails, use a wash cloth moistened with a weak shampoo and water solution. Put a towel under her head. Remember the plastic bag mentioned earlier? It can come in very handy here, under the towel.

WRITE NOTES HERE

CHAPTER 5

SHAVING

WARNING: IF ALICE IS A DIABETIC OR TAKES A BLOOD THINNER, BLADE SHAVING IS NOT ADVISABLE.

A cut on a diabetic's leg can quickly become a large sore. If Alice is on a blood thinner such as Coumadin, a tiny nick can bleed profusely and not heal. If you are uncertain about what Alice's medicine is and what it does, contact his physician, nurse or pharmacist.

A FEW MORE WORDS OF WARNING: IF ALICE IS ON OXYGEN THERAPY DON'T USE AN ELECTRIC RAZOR.

If you do, Alice should turn off her oxygen and remove the *cannula,* the tubing he/she wears on her face. If the razor has a cord it can pull loose possibly causing sparks. These sparks can cause the oxygen to ignite, burning Alice. Even rechargeable razors can pose a risk. Alice should not remove the cannula and set it aside, leaving the oxygen flow on; it could still ignite.

Several years ago a patient insisted on smoking while on oxygen therapy, despite being warned of the hazards. The oxygen ignited. He received severe burns to the face, nose, lips and neck. Worse, he suffered severe internal burns as well. *It is important to follow all operational directions and hazard warnings when caring for Alice at home!*

Ladies First

BLADE SHAVING

After a bath is a good time for Alice to shave her legs because the hairs are softer and can be shaved off with less likelihood of skin irritation. If she is able to take a shower or tub bath, do the shaving there. These directions are for shaving Alice's legs in bed.

PREPARATION

Collect the necessary paraphernalia, including gloves. *(You didn't forget those gloves, did you?)*

Spread that ever present towel under Alice's legs. Dip a clean washcloth in a basin of warm water and moisten the area to be shaved. Work in sections so Alice doesn't freeze. For example, do the front of the lower leg, then the back, then the upper front and so on. Whatever is not being shaved should be covered.

HOW TO DO IT – STEP-BY-STEP

1. Wet the skin and spread some lotion before applying shaving foam/gel. The lotion adds extra lubrication and makes the experience more comfortable for Alice. It also prevents excessive drying of the skin. Lotion tends to build up on the razor so rinse often and rinse well.

2. Use a generous amount of foam or gel. Make sure the razor isn't dull, clogged or rusty. Wet it well before starting. If Alice is able, let her do the actual shaving. If she can't, use a light touch. Think about how you shave. Use long smooth strokes rather than short choppy ones.

3. Start from the ankles and work your way up. If Alice shaves herself, she also should work her way up, so that the more tired she gets, the less she will be bending or reaching. This reduces the chance of Alice getting dizzy while bending over - which reduces her risk of falling. If she tires out completely and can't finish, at least the more visible portions - the calves - will be done. She can always do more with tomorrow's bath!

4. Rinse thoroughly with a washcloth. Apply a skin soother if desired. Aloe works well. Wait a while before applying more lotion - shaving causes tiny nicks and opens up skin pores. Lotion can clog these pores and irritate the nicks.

For Women with Whiskers

It's a fact of life that some women develop facial hair as they age. The occasional hair can be plucked with tweezers. Wash Alice's face with warm water and soap, then dry gently. This will open pores making tweezing easier. Be sure the tweezers are clean. Consider shaving if plucking doesn't work. The technique is the same as for men except women's whiskers are usually softer. If there aren't whiskers growing in an area, don't shave it.

Now for the Gentlemen

BLADE SHAVING

Collect your supplies, including gloves. Drape a towel around Mr. Alice's neck, covering his chest. Wash his face if he hasn't already done so during his bath. Soak his beard for a few minutes with a very warm, moist washcloth. Apply lotion, then shaving cream.

Pay attention to the direction Alice's whiskers grow. Most men shave their face in a downward motion, angling slightly forward. Take special care around the nose, mouth, and ears. He should be able to assist you by making various facial contortions - opening his mouth or bulging his cheek out with his tongue.

Usually, the neck area is shaved with longer, upward strokes. Be careful, Alice's skin is thinner here. Have Alice raise his head to tighten the skin of his neck. Pivoting razors are really a big help here.

His and Hers

UNDERARMS

In some instances, it may be necessary for men to shave their underarms. Deodorants, and medications for rashes, are easier to apply with underarm hair removed, thus making them more effective.

For long growth, carefully trim with scissors. For blade shaving, wash with soap and warm water, then apply a non-irritating shave foam or gel. Underarm skin is very tender and easily gets razor burn, so use a light touch with only a few strokes. Shaving in the direction of hair growth prevents irritation.

ELECTRIC RAZORS

Many men and women prefer the ease and convenience of electric razors. Shaving can be done virtually anytime.

Pre-shave preparations are available to make hair/whiskers stand up and to help the razor slide more easily over the skin. An economical option is baby powder, if Alice doesn't have any breathing complications. The powder helps reduce friction, thereby reducing razor drag and rash.

Use a light touch, especially if electric shaving is a new experience for you or Alice. Be sure to clean the razor according to the manufacturer's instructions. Avoid wiping or brushing over the screen or blades; this dulls blades and can break the screen.

As usual, gather those supplies first. Spread out a towel to ease clean-up. Make sure Alice's skin is clean and dry.

What if blade shaving is a no-no but Alice isn't happy with the results from an electric razor? Consider a wet/dry electric. They perform much better than conventional electric razors. Remember to use a light touch, especially the first few times - the razor can cause irritation until Alice becomes accustomed to it. Don't be discouraged if the shave is not very close the first few times you use an electric razor. Results improve with repeated use and practice. Electric shavers are available for men and women.

CHAPTER 6

AVOIDING SKIN IRRITATION: THE POWER OF CORN STARCH

Anyone who has ever cared for a baby knows that dry skin is healthy skin. Even if Alice does not have bladder control problems, known as *urinary incontinence,* she may develop diaper rash from perspiration. Other moisture prone areas under breasts, arms and abdominal skin folds can become rashy as well.

Corn starch can prevent these skin irritations. After Alice bathes, dust a light layer of corn starch onto moisture prone areas. Use a powder puff or folded washcloth to apply - like powder, corn starch can be an irritant to people with breathing difficulty. Make sure Alice's skin is dry before applying.

For a fresher fragrance, mix the corn starch with regular talcum or dusting powder. About half and half works well. This mixture can be stored in a recycled butter tub. Or, if Alice prefers to sprinkle the powder herself, recycle a shaker top plastic spice bottle with smallish holes. Just wash the bottle well and allow it to dry thoroughly before using. You might consider putting a label on it, just to be on the safe side – the talcum might give your next batch of batter dipped pork chops a rather "unusual" taste. By the way, you can also use a spice bottle for corn starch in the kitchen. Those little boxes with the bags inside are such a pain, aren't they?

Incontinence, and medications which cause excessive sweating, are common causes of excessive moisture which could cause powders or corn starch to become a wet sticky mess, leading to skin irritation and bacterial growth in thigh or buttock creases. If this occurs try switching to a light layer of petroleum jelly in the creases of the upper thighs and buttocks (diaper area). The jelly can even be used under breasts or arms. If you use jelly, do not use also use powder or corn starch due to the possibility of bacterial growth.

If Alice is a diabetic, her urine may be rich in sugar. Excess sugar in the urine provides food for bacteria, causing her to be especially prone to skin irritation, and bladder and vaginal yeast infections. Be especially conscious of Alice's skin care needs. Observe her skin closely for signs of irritation or breakdown. It is especially important to keep her skin clear, dry, and whole because it is often difficult for diabetics to heal.

CHAPTER 7

BACK RUBS

Alice tells me that nothing is more soothing than a back rub. They are especially relaxing if she can't get out of bed or if she spends many hours in a chair. Back rubs can increase circulation and relax muscles.

Alice may have dry or even flaky skin on her back. A massage with lotion or oil can help to moisturize.

WARNING! CHECK WITH ALICE'S PHYSICIAN OR HOME HEALTH NURSE TO FIND OUT IF SHE EVER HAD A BACK INJURY. USE A VERY LIGHT TOUCH IF SHE HAS BEEN DIAGNOSED WITH *OSTEOPOROSIS* (BRITTLE BONES).

To make massage a comfortable experience, warm the lotion or oil in a basin of warm water or in the microwave. If you do zap it, make sure the cap is open. Don't put a tube of lotion in the microwave. Better yet, warm some in a saucer or small bowl. Zap it for a few seconds at a time, to avoid overheating and splattering.

Alice may like to have her back rubbed after her bath, before she puts on her blouse. Or she may prefer to have it done later, after she has rested. Alice may prefer powder or lotion when she gets her back rubbed. She might complain of feeling sticky after using lotion. Try a light dusting of powder afterwards to counteract the stickiness. Remember to use a powder puff, don't shake.

Gather all your materials - powder, lotion, towel. . . Police the area to ensure privacy and warmth. Remember to remove rings, watches and other jewelry first. Back rubs can be given with or without gloves. I prefer to wear them; lotion coats the gloves allowing them to slide over Alice's skin more easily. Alice can sit up in bed or a chair, lie on her stomach or on her side. Choose a position comfortable for both of you. No sense in giving *Alice* a back rub if it is going to give *you* a back ache.

Massaging is surprisingly similar to kneading bread dough. You can massage flat handed or use the heels of your hands and the sides of your thumbs to relax Alice's muscles. Don't use your fingertips - it doesn't feel good. As you massage, think about the structure of the muscles. *See Figure J*

Rub along the length of the muscles. Your goal is to limber them and stretch them out. If you want to stretch out a length of elastic *(which is essentially what a muscle is)* you stretch it lengthwise, not side to side. Work along the length of the muscle groups. Start with the neck and shoulders. Work the muscles on the back of her shoulders, moving the pads of the thumbs in a circular motion. Remember, don't use your fingertips, the pinching motion created is not usually considered relaxing. Start close to the neck and progress toward the shoulders. Work up the neck with the flat part of the fingers.

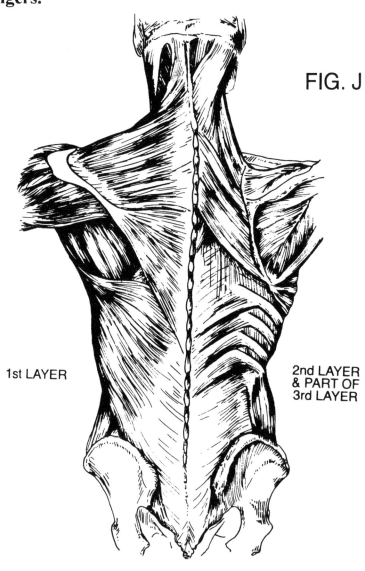

FIG. J

1st LAYER

2nd LAYER
& PART OF
3rd LAYER

Now for Alice's back. Use the heels and palms of your hands. Alternate long, smooth strokes with a series of circles using your thumbs or the heels of your hands. Start from the waist and work up. Concentrate on the muscles along the spine. Encourage Alice to give you feedback on how you are doing. If she can't, you can still give her back rubs. Just be extra gentle to avoid any injury.

If you wind up with too much lotion, simply blot it off with a small towel. Cover areas you are not working on with a towel or sheet. This protects Alice's privacy and it keeps her warm.

Back rubs can be given through a t-shirt or blouse. You can put powder on under her shirt. Just skip the lotion or use it sparingly. Unhook her bra so you don't rub the straps into Alice's back.

WRITE NOTES HERE

CHAPTER 8
MOUTH CARE

Alice should brush her teeth at least twice a day. If she is able to get up and walk to the bathroom, Alice should be brushing pretty well on her own. However, if Alice has an illness such as Alzheimer's, she will probably require your supervision to guarantee thorough and safe brushing. We'll talk more about that in just a little bit.

Meanwhile, let's talk about brushing Alice's teeth if she is bed or chair bound.

PREPARATION

First? Right! Gather those supplies. You will need toothpaste, a brush, a cup of water and something for Alice to spit in. A plastic wash basin is good, it provides a large target. Did you remember to wash your hands? Gloves? If you have to actively participate in the brushing process, it's a good idea to put them on.

Wet the brush, apply some toothpaste, and brush. Be gentle but thorough. Think about how you brush your own teeth. Brush for at least two minutes *(those little hour glass egg timers are a great way to keep track of brushing time).* Rinse well.

The latest crazes in mouth care seem to be tartar control and peroxide toothpastes. Some individuals find tartar control pastes too harsh, reporting blisters on their gums after regular use. Consider alternating with milder paste to produce the extra cleansing action without the painful side effects.

When peroxide is used for wound care, it is important not to leave it on too long. Peroxide does not discriminate between infected and healthy tissue; it destroys them both. Let us hope the concentration of peroxide in toothpaste is weak enough to make this a non-issue, but is the effect cumulative? Does peroxide speed up the process of wearing it away? The enamel on Alice's teeth is not going to replace itself. If Alice really wants the extra cleaning action of peroxide, buy a fifty cent bottle of hydrogen peroxide with which to rinse her mouth periodically. It's a lot cheaper and directions are on the bottle.

Flossing is important too. If Alice is unable to do it herself, get a floss holder or disposable floss wands. These eliminate the need to stick both hands in Alice's mouth – like she'd even let you!

Periodically soak Alice's brush in hydrogen peroxide or a mixture of peroxide and mouthwash. Rinse well before using. This will sanitize the brush. Replace brushes when worn – about every three months.

For patients with learning deficits and illnesses such as Alzheimer's, bright and colorful children's brushes may make the experience more pleasant. Electric varieties are also effective; consider a rechargeable brush so there are no dangling cords to worry about. Children's toothpaste comes in flavors ranging from fruit to bubble gum. These flavors may encourage a reluctant brusher to be more cooperative.

Try to prevent Alice from swallowing the toothpaste – which is very possible if she suffers from an illness such as Alzheimer's. Also, be wary of getting bitten by Alice – it *HURTS!*

SORES AND FUNGAL INFECTIONS

Examine Alice's mouth for sores and other problems. If she has been on antibiotics, she can develop a fungal infection known as *thrush,* which usually occurs when antibiotics kill off good bacteria, allowing bad bacteria to flourish. Another cause is poor oral hygiene. Signs of thrush are the appearance of thick white patches and reddened areas. Alice may complain of mouth pain, especially when eating or drinking. If she is unable to communicate, a decrease is appetite and drooling could be indications of thrush.

Prescription mouth rinses are available to treat thrush, but first try plain yogurt with active culture; it restores the natural bacteria necessary for a healthy mouth and digestive tract. It helps for Alice just to eat the yogurt. For better results she should swish it around in her mouth before swallowing. Try to avoid the sweetened, fruity varieties unless they are the only kind Alice will tolerate.

DENTURES

If Alice has dentures take them out and soak or brush them. There are many cleansers available; just follow the package directions. Always clean out Alice's mouth at least once, and preferably, twice, a day. A clean, wet washcloth or a soft brush with a dab of toothpaste works well. If a home health nurse visits Alice the nurse may be able to supply her with sponge swabs designed for cleaning the mouth. These can be used with toothpaste or mouthwash. Check the baby care section of your store for preparations to remove plaque from teeth and gums.

Check Alice's dentures for proper fit. Bones and gums shrink as we age; dentures don't. Poorly fitting dentures are uncomfortable and embarrassing; they make speech and chewing difficult. Trying to fill gaps with goop and adhesives is only a temporary solution.

Encourage Alice to keep her dentures in when she is awake. This may prevent further gum shrinkage and keeps her gums accustomed to the dentures. It is especially *not* recommended to sleep *(note: napping is sleeping!)* with partials in place; they might accidentally be swallowed. This seemingly innocent habit could prove to be fatal.

Clean Alice's dentures and store them in a denture holder. Don't soak them all night, just rinse them off before she puts them back in.

DENTAL CHECKUPS

Whether Alice has her own teeth or wears dentures, regular dental checkups are still important. I have been told that some dentists even make house calls. If Alice is unable to travel, contact her dentist to see if a house call is an option. Also, contact Alice's insurance company to determine if house calls are covered. If they are covered, the insurance company should be able to provide the names and telephone numbers of dentists willing to provide this service.

WRITE NOTES HERE

CHAPTER 9

EAR CARE

Ever read the warning on a box of cotton swabs? *"Do not insert swab into ear canal."* I know, I know. I do it, too.

But you really shouldn't when it comes to caring for Alice. Why risk puncturing Alice's ear drum? Besides, trying to remove wax with a swab doesn't really work; it just pushes most of it back into her ear.

Instead, use inexpensive drops which are available in many stores. The drops soften the ear wax and bubble it to the outer ear where it can be wiped away with a damp cloth. Speak with Alice's physician or nurse if her ears are really full of wax. Do not use these drops if Alice has an ear infection. Indications of infection are pain, swelling, drainage and foul odor from Alice's ear.

The outer portion of the ear also needs to be clean. Check the skin behind Alice's ears. It should be clean, dry and intact. It's an area which is often overlooked and it can easily become crusty and irritated.

Ears are an important area to watch if Alice is bed bound and can't move around on her own. If she lies on her side too long, reddened areas can form on her ear. If ignored, she can develop pressure sores *(decubitus ulcers)*. Reposition Alice every two hours if she cannot turn herself. Turn her from one side to the other, or onto her back.

If Alice wears oxygen tubing she will probably develop sore ears. To relieve, or even prevent, soreness the tubing can be padded with tissue or gauze. The little sponge end wraps from some home perm kits are also good padding - just secure them with a little soft bandage tape. Be very careful not to step on the tubing while Alice walks or moves around.

Time for another true story. A patient's wife stepped on his oxygen tubing when he stood up. The tubing is very strong plastic. It didn't break. His skin did - his ear was torn nearly halfway through. Know where the tubing is when you are working with Alice. It may have a clip to attach it to Alice's clothing. If it does not, consider using a large safety pin or a diaper pin. Don't pin through the tubing, just around it.

WRITE NOTES HERE

CHAPTER 10

NASAL CARE

You probably didn't think about taking care of Alice's nose, did you? Even if she is able to blow her nose herself, there are other factors to consider. This is especially true if she is on oxygen therapy or medications which cause the nasal passages to dry out.

Just like skin, mucous membranes can be lubricated. Don't lubricate with any petroleum based ointments or lotions, though. Instead, use a water soluble lubricant such as KY Jelly®. Generics are fine. Apply with a clean, gloved fingertip or cotton swab.

What's wrong with lotions or petroleum jelly?

Both are oil based. Tiny droplets of oil are inhaled if these are used in the nose. These droplets end up coating the lungs and interfere with oxygen absorption. Not good no matter what your age. Check with Alice's physician about ocean sprays. These weak saltwater sprays are available almost anywhere and can help moisturize the nose.

CHAPTER 11

URINARY INCONTINENCE: WHAT IT IS. WHAT TO DO.

Urinary incontinence is the loss of bladder control. Many times I have heard little old ladies say they can't control their kidneys. No one can. Most of us can control our bladder, however.

Causes of incontinence include: childbirth, stroke, bladder cancer, medications, infections, general aging and even surgery (for example, many men who undergo prostate surgery experience some degree of incontinence).

Not only is incontinence inconvenient and embarrassing, but it causes the skin to be continually moist, allowing bacteria to grow, causing skin breakdown. Urine, plus the ammonia and other materials which form when urine decomposes, are also irritating to the skin.

TO HELP REGAIN CONTROL

Limit fluids after 6 p.m. or however necessary to prevent nighttime accidents. *Do not* limit fluids if Alice is on any type of fluid restriction or forced fluid treatment, as is common with certain heart ailments and medications. Always consult Alice's physician or home health nurse first.

There are exercises to help Alice regain control. The most effective are called Kegel exercises. Alice tightens her buttock and groin muscles, as if trying not to urinate. She relaxes, then flexes again, repeating a total of ten times. It may be awhile before she can do this ten consecutive times.

Alice should do Kegel exercises 3-4 times a day. Kegels are easy and can be done anywhere. Actually, they are good for all of us - they help muscle tone and are even rumored to improve your sex life!

Another exercise can be performed when Alice urinates. Using muscle control, she stops the stream of urine, starts it again, stops it and so on. At first this is difficult, if not impossible. With practice it is easier and can be very effective. If Alice loses control only in physical stress situations *(standing, sneezing, climbing steps . . .)* these exercises should be especially helpful.

Establish a regular schedule or routine for Alice to use the bathroom. For example, accidents may be reduced by making a habit of taking Alice to the bathroom when she wakes up, plus several times during the day, and again at bedtime. Never wait until Alice has "to go" desperately. Waiting to urinate is bad for anyone. It promotes bladder infections and damages the bladder. Signs of bladder infection are urgency, increased frequency, or painful urination, as well as blood or mucus in the urine. If any of these symptoms is noted, Alice should be checked for a bladder infection.

If Alice can get up, but doesn't walk well consider getting a bedside commode. These are also helpful if she has "to go" during the night. If she is bedfast, bedpans are an option. Plastic ones aren't as cold as the infamous stainless steel pans. If a regular pan is too big and uncomfortable, a wedge shaped fracture pan may prove to be more comfortable. These were designed for patients with hip-fractures. Beware. They do not hold very much!

Both styles are illustrated in *Figure K* Bedpans can be bought at medical supply stores and hospitals (the central supply division). Many home health catalogs carry them as well.

FIG. K

WHEN REGAINING CONTROL IS NOT AN OPTION

When nothing else works, or if Alice is afflicted with a condition such as advanced Alzheimer's and cannot tell you when she needs to go, Alice – and her surroundings – need to be protected with a urine-absorbing material.

As a result of the recent development of materials that gel when wet, protective products have become smaller and more absorbent than those used 10 or more years ago. Everything from small pads, which resemble feminine napkins, to adult size diapers, are now available at your local supermarket.

Disposable waterproof pads can be used on beds and chairs. It is advisable to have one of these pads under Alice if she is a bedpan patron. Nursing homes use a washable quilted pad with a rubber backing. Look in the baby section of the department store for rubber pads. Medical supply stores carry many types of pads and supplies.

Regardless of what manner of protection is used, be sure it is changed as soon as possible once it becomes wet; this will prevent skin breakdown, and will make Alice more comfortable. Resist the temptation to dry disposable pads and reuse them. Even after they are dry, the residue from the urine can still irritate the skin.

How do you get a diaper on Alice if she can't get out of bed? In the situation where she needs it the most, it's the hardest to do. It's not like diapering a baby.

If Alice is able - and willing - to turn, it's really pretty easy. If not - maybe Alice is one of those patients who always seems to slide down to the foot of the bed and cannot push herself back up to the top - using a *draw sheet* still makes it possible. A draw sheet can be used to turn Alice from side to side and even pull her up in the bed.

A draw sheet can be improvised by folding a flat sheet in half, hems together. It is positioned underneath Alice, with the top folded edge underneath her neck. The bottom edge should reach to about mid-thigh. The edges should hang over the sides of the bed. See Figure L

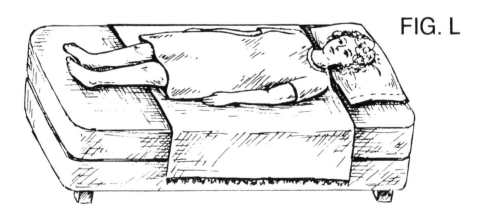

FIG. L

I'll explain how to use the draw sheet in just a few minutes.

PREPARATION

For now, let's assume Alice just came home from the hospital and her diaper is full. Of everything. She's on her back, with the head of the bed raised and she cannot move independently. You read this book before she came home, so the draw sheet is already on the bed. We'll talk about changing the draw sheet and the soiled bedclothes a little later.

Assemble your supplies: a trash bag or waste receptacle, clean diaper, basin of water, washcloths, baby wipes or tissue, soap, petroleum jelly and – of course - gloves. Powder or corn starch are optional. I prefer straight petroleum jelly, having survived the diaper rash prevention scene with my son. It's cheap and it works. Powder and corn starch are breeding grounds for bacteria when very moist.

HOW TO DO IT- STEP-BY-STEP

1. Lower the head of the bed. Have Alice bend her knees and raise her hips. Help her if she can't do it herself. Slip a towel underneath her hips to help protect the bed. Straighten her legs and move her feet apart.

2. Unfasten the diaper and roll the front of it down and to the inside. Pull it down so the groin area is exposed. If stool has worked around to the front of the diaper, use tissue, baby wipes or white bleach proof cloths to wipe it away. Wet and

soap a washcloth and squeeze it out over the groin area. Do this several times, until clean.

3. Wash and rinse the area well. Dry well but gently. Apply a thin layer of petroleum jelly to creases at tops of thighs. This area is often prone to moisture irritation.

USING A DRAW SHEET TO TURN ALICE

4. Now for the draw sheet. There are two ways it can be used.

   A) Stand at the bedside, roughly at Alice's waist level. If she has a hospital bed, first lower the foot end of the rail. Leave the head end up unless it blocks your reach. Alice can hold on to the rail as she turns. Reach across to the opposite side of the bed and grasp the side edges of the draw sheet. *See Figure M1* Pull toward you, as shown in *Figure M2* This makes a sling under Alice. As she rolls toward you, be sure there is room for her to turn.

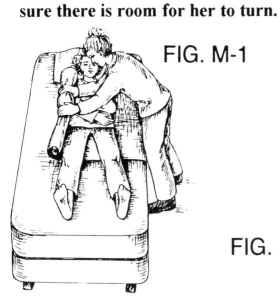

FIG. M-1

FIG. M-2

B) Position yourself at the bedside, at Alice's waist level. Grasp the side edges of the draw sheet on the same side of the bed as you are on. Pull toward yourself, slightly upward. It might help to roll the edge of the sheet like a jelly roll first, for a better grip. See Figures N1 and N2

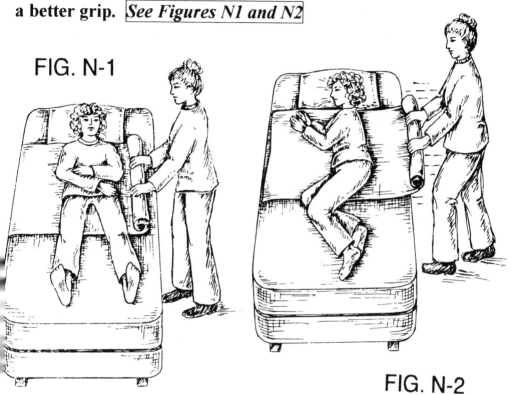

FIG. N-1

FIG. N-2

This should roll Alice in place as the sheet feeds through beneath her. It is not the most comfortable way for Alice to be turned. And it takes quite a bit of effort until you get the hang of it. But it makes the impossible, possible, and can be done by one person. I'm 5'1" and weigh around 110 pounds *(depending on how close to the holidays we are)*. I spent 5+ years turning people with this method . . . and some of my patients topped 300 pounds. It *will* work!

4. Sometimes it takes a combination of both methods to turn Alice. Once you get her turned over, straighten out the draw sheet. Spread a large towel under Alice's buttock area. Tuck it under her to keep the bed dry. In a moment we'll explain how a similar technique can allow you to change the bed with Alice in it.

5. Now, open the back of the diaper and roll it toward Alice, jelly roll style. Roll it to the inside, so the waterproof plastic outside is exposed. Pull the rolled front portion of the diaper from between Alice's legs. Wipe buttocks and anal area with tissue, baby wipes or white cloths. Wash Alice's buttocks and anal area with a soapy wash cloth and rinse well. Pat dry. Apply a thin layer petroleum jelly to buttocks and anal area.

6. Look for reddened, raw areas. Sadly, patients often come home from the hospital or nursing home with them. Stage II decubitus *(See Chapter 13: Decubitis Ulcers: Prevention & Treatment)* or worse needs attention from Alice's doctor or home health nurse (Stage I decubitus will usually resolve itself once pressure is relieved). In the meantime, keep the affected areas clean and dry. Don't put any medication or powder on them. And don't massage them! (Massage was SOP – *Standard Operating Procedure* – for many years until a relatively recent discovery that massage was actually harmful.)

7. Now Alice is clean. How to get a clean diaper on her and get rid of this other one? Open a clean diaper. Roll or fold the back portion lengthwise to almost halfway. *See Figure O* Position the back of the diaper against Alice's backside, next to the soiled diaper. *See Figure P1* Pull the front of the soiled diaper back between her thighs. Roll up the towel. It should wind up next to the clean diaper. Using the draw sheet, turn Alice onto her back, then over to her other side.

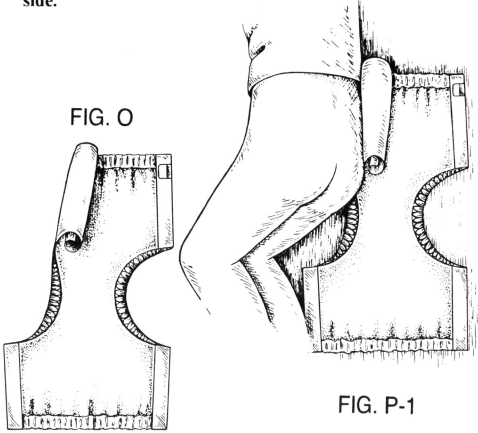

FIG. O

FIG. P-1

8. Carefully remove the old diaper. With a clean cloth, wash Alice's other hip, then her buttock. Massage in petroleum jelly. Make note of any decubitus ulcers and treat as in (7) above. Remove the towel. Unroll the back of the clean diaper and spread it out. *See Figure P2*

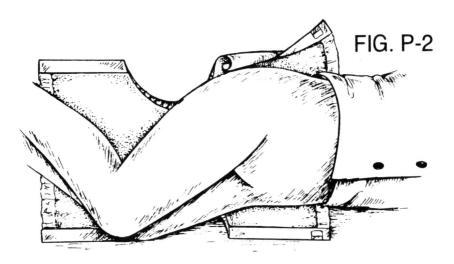

FIG. P-2

9. Turn Alice onto her back. Adjust the front of the diaper and fasten the tapes. Make sure they are straight and don't poke into Alice's skin. With practice, you can tell where to position the diaper so it ends up in the right place on the first try.

10. Be careful not to get lotion or powder on the tapes; either will keep them from sticking. Because that *will* happen, sooner or later, keep a couple of diaper pins on hand. Open the tapes, put them in place, then pin right through them.

Uh-oh. You tore the diaper during all that turning and unrolling. No problem. Mend it with cellophane or masking tape, or that two inch wide box packing tape.

OTHER USES OF THE DRAW SHEET

How do you use a draw sheet to pull Alice up in bed?

     Two People: Stand one on each side of the bed. Roll up the edges of the draw sheet for a better grip. Lift and slide toward the head of the bed. Use your legs not your back. *See Figure Q*

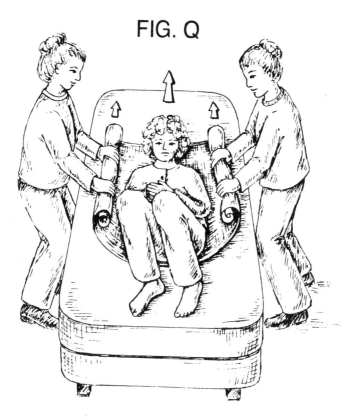

FIG. Q

One Person: Stand at the head of the bed. Grasp the draw sheet, roll it a little, on either side of Alice's head near her shoulders. Brace your thighs or stomach on the bed. Height makes a difference here. Pull to you. Remember to use your legs not your back. See Figure R

FIG. R

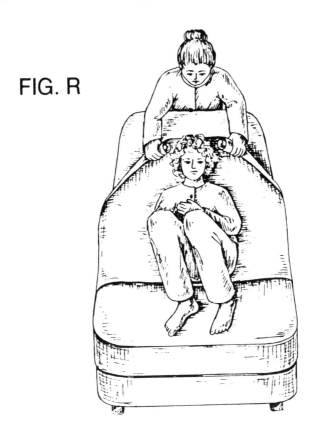

To change an occupied bed, turn Alice with the draw sheet. Loosen the bedclothes on the side behind Alice and jelly roll them toward her back, including the draw sheet. Put that side of the clean bedclothes on, rolling the remaining side the same way, leaving it next to the soiled linens. Put on a bottom sheet, draw sheet and waterproof pads, if needed.

Cross to the other side. Turn Alice using the draw sheet. If it pulls out, turn her with gentle pressure on her hip and shoulder. Roll her over the jelly rolls of linens. Remove the soiled bed clothes. Unroll the clean linens a layer at a time and finish making the bed.

This is a good time to point out that regular twin sheets don't fit most hospital beds. Full sized flat sheets don't stay on either, do they? They do if you tie them on. Here's how you do that.

Starting at the head of the bed, raise the mattress - prop it on your knee or even the top of your head - and tie the two upper corners of the sheet together under the mattress. Lower the mattress and do the same at the foot. When you lower the foot of the mattress, its weight should pull the sheet nice and tight. No wrinkles to produce lines and sore spots on Alice's skin. With practice it's quick and effective. Just don't try it with Alice in the bed, unless she's an adventurous sort . . . and you're very strong!

WRITE NOTES HERE

CHAPTER 12

CATHETER CARE

Even though Alice had a catheter while she was in the hospital, you never expected her to come home with one.

There it is. She's embarrassed. You're embarrassed. Who is going to take care of it? Chances are, if you're reading this book, it's going to be *you!*

What is a catheter?

It's a tube inserted in the bladder to drain urine. It is held in place by a small balloon inflated after the catheter is inserted. *See Figure S1*

Why does Alice need one?

Maybe Alice had a stroke, or cancer or bladder surgery. Any of these, plus many other causes, have left Alice unable to empty her bladder normally. Perhaps there is a need to maintain an empty bladder to avoid pressure - following surgery, for instance.

FIG. S-1

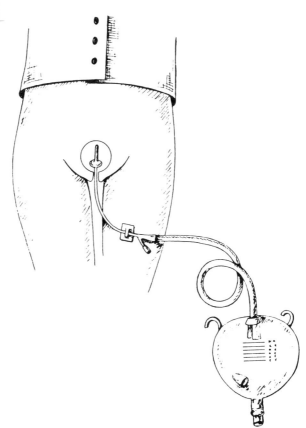

How do you take care of it?

One of the most important rules is to keep it attached to her leg with tape, a strap or a tubing anchor. A nearby hospital central supply division or a home health supply store can probably help you locate these.

You should be aware that some tapes cause skin irritation. Be on the lookout for redness, blistering, or peeling skin. Change the tape every day, placing it in a slightly different location to avoid irritation.

The catheter tubing should be anchored so when Alice bends or stands, there isn't be any tension on the catheter. Tension is not only uncomfortable, it can pull the catheter out. *Ouch!*

The clear tubing leading from the catheter to the drainage bag should be coiled, with no kinks or twists. The bag should always remain below the level of the bladder to facilitate drainage. Urine should not back up in the tubing - it will re-enter the bladder and can cause infection. Under normal circumstances the inside of Alice's bladder is sterile. So is her urine. After it reaches the drainage bag, it begins to break down *(decompose)*. The bag does not remain sterile.

How do you give Alice a bath when she's "wearing" this thing? If she can take a shower the only major concern is avoiding tension on the tubing. I wouldn't recommend tub baths - where could you put the drainage bag so it will be lower than Alice's bladder when she is in the tub? Probably nowhere – which means that urine could travel back up the tube to her bladder and possibly cause infection.

Most likely Alice will be taking bed baths. Washing the genital area is still pretty much the same as we discussed earlier in *Chapter 2: Personal Care & Bathing,* but with some special precautions because of the catheter. Are you ready? Well, you already know the first step: find your gloves and assemble the supplies.

HOW TO DO IT – STEP-BY-STEP

1. First wash around the catheter, being careful not to dislodge it.

2. Now wash the catheter. Begin with the part closest to Alice. Hold the catheter with your free hand to keep from pulling it out. Fold the washcloth loosely over the catheter and wipe down its length. Rinse in the same fashion.

3. Now wash the surrounding area, taking care to always wash the genital area before the anal area.

O.K. You've put it off as long as you can. Alice's drainage bag needs to be emptied. Her doctor wants you to keep track of how much urine she passes every 24 hours. A container with markings to measure, usually in c.c.'s - cubic centimeters - should have been sent home with Alice. How do you do this? That's the next procedure we'll explain.

Note that if records of Alice's urine output are not required, *you'll still need to follow the procedure below.* You can empty her catheter bag into a clean container reserved specifically for that purpose (the bucket from a bedside commode works quite well for this, as do large plastic pitchers with handles), then dispose of the contents in the toilet. While almost any clean container will do the job, I prefer one with handles. They guarantee a good grip ... and that prevents spills, a desirable thing when working with someone else's bodily wastes!

HOW TO DO IT – STEP-BY-STEP

1. First, wash your hands, preferably with an antibacterial soap. Don't forget: GLOVES, *GLOVES*, *GLOVES!*

2. There is a valve at the bottom of the drainage bag with a clamp on it. Position the clean container under the valve and open the clamp SLOWLY. Nothing quite ruins your day like getting splashed in the face with someone else's urine. Don't let the valve touch the container. Don't let the urine in the container touch the valve. Remember, every time you open the bag you risk introducing bacteria into the system. These bacteria can travel through the catheter into Alice's bladder and even up into her kidneys to cause a serious, perhaps even life-threatening, infection.

3. Close the valve. Some physicians advise wiping the valve with an alcohol wipe, some don't. Ask Alice's physician or home health nurse about their policy on this.

4. Record the amount of urine drained, the date and time. While this may not be required, it's not a bad habit. You may have to empty the container a couple of times. Be sure to drain the bag completely. Rinse the container with water and disinfectant after each case. Do not use bleach to clean

the container; it can combine with the ammonia that forms from urine breakdown, to produce a toxic gas.

While you are up close and personal with Alice's urine, check for signs of a UTI (urinary tract infection). The most common are: cloudy urine (resulting from mucous formation) and blood in the urine. Another sign – Alice complains of pain or spasms in the bladder region. Although a catheter is not a joy to wear it should be bearable. Excess discomfort usually indicates a problem.

How does Alice walk around, get out of the house, or travel while she is wearing her catheter? She may be able to use a device known as a leg bag. *See Figure S2*

This bag attaches to the catheter, without the clear tubing. It should only be worn when Alice is up on her feet or sitting up. It is not advisable to use a leg bag if she sits in a recliner. If she wears it when lying down, urine will drain back into her bladder, possibly causing an infection.

The advantage of a leg bag is it can be concealed under a dress, gown or slacks. The disadvantages are they don't hold as much and therefore must be emptied more often. And that Alice might find the straps which are attached to the bag to be uncomfortable.

Don't remove the clear drainage tubing from the catheter, or attempt to attach a leg bag to the catheter without being carefully instructed on how to do so, in person, by a home health care practitioner. With the exception of the valve that drains the bag, this is a closed and sterile system. Opening it anywhere except at the drainage valve dramatically increases the risk of infection.

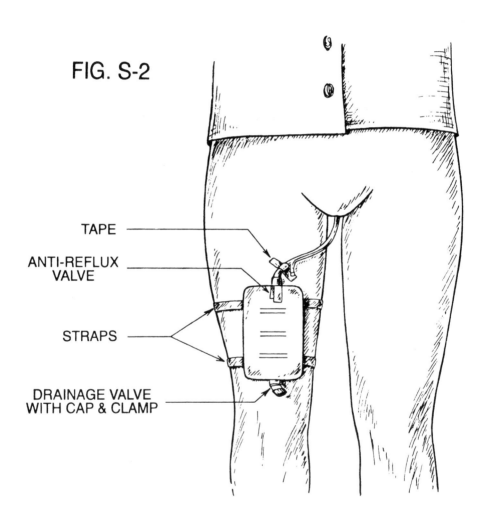

FIG. S-2

TAPE

ANTI-REFLUX VALVE

STRAPS

DRAINAGE VALVE WITH CAP & CLAMP

CHAPTER 13

DECUBITUS ULCERS: PREVENTION & TREATMENT

Perhaps the worst enemy of the bedridden are *decubitus ulcers,* commonly referred to as *bed sores.* These occur when tissue covering bony prominences - such as hip bones, shoulder blades, heels, elbows, and even ears - are in constant contact with, and under pressure from, a mattress, chair, pillow or even another body part.

As a result of the pressure, blood circulation to the skin in that area is reduced or ceases. Without sufficient circulating blood – which supplies oxygen and vital nutrients, and removes waste products - the skin begins to die. Wheelchairs, catheter tubes, and other objects which continually rub against the skin can produce the same problem. Bed and chair bound patients are particularly at risk.

The Condition & Treatment

The severity of the decubitus is described using a rating system of Roman numerals. There are five stages of decubitus, designated Stages I through V, though Stage V is only rarely found. The larger the number, the greater the severity.

STAGE I DECUBITIS

Stage I is easily recognized as reddened, unbroken skin. It quickly disappears when the source of the pressure is removed. Treatment involves repositioning or providing additional padding or cushions to remove pressure. Do not use donut cushions - these concentrate pressure in a smaller area. They also restrict circulation to the area inside the center opening.

Former treatment methods included massage of reddened areas. Health professionals now realize that massage creates friction or shearing, increasing skin injury; so massage is *not* to be used.

If at all possible, Alice's nutritional intake should be increased to promote *healing*. Proteins, vitamin C and fluids are especially important. Good nutrition also helps *prevent* skin breakdown.

STAGE II DECUBITIS

In Stage II decubitus, a blister forms over the top of the reddened area. The blister may be broken or filled with fluid.

Caring for a Stage II case involves keeping it clean, covered and protected from any additional pressure. Dressings should be absorbent and provide padding.

If treated quickly, a Stage II case can heal rapidly. If left untreated, a Stage II can quickly become a Stage III, which is worse and harder to heal.

STAGE III DECUBITIS

Stage III extends through all layers of skin tissue. It provides an entrance for bacteria and other infectious organisms.

Treatment of a Stage III case is essentially the same as that of a Stage II; keeping it clean and using absorbent, protective padding. Nutrient and fluid intake should be increased to promote healing. Without proper nutrition and care, the stage III will quickly progress to a Stage IV.

STAGE IV DECUBITIS

Stage IV decubitus involve all layers of the skin, plus underlying tissue, bone, tendon, and muscle. Proper nutrition and fluid intake are essential or these wounds will not heal. Wound treatment remains the same as for Stage III – keep the wound clean, dry and well protected.

The appearance of a Stage IV wound can be deceptive. The depth of the wound is more important than the diameter. Decubitus of this severity is life threatening and if Alice has developed a Stage IV case, she needs immediate medical care by a medical practitioner trained in wound care. In some cases, *debridement* (removal of the dead tissue) is needed before healing can begin.

WARNING: DO NOT ATTEMPT TO TREAT STAGE IV DECUBITIS. SEEK IMMEDIATE MEDICAL HELP.

STAGE V DECUBITIS

In some cases, decubitus may be rated as stage V. These are extremely deep, extending into bones, organs and muscles. Healing rarely occurs. Treatment usually involves surgical debridement. Frequent dressing changes are usually necessary as these wounds usually have a significant amount of drainage.

Prevention

The most effective way to treat decubitus is to prevent it. Alice should change positions at least every two hours. If Alice can't turn herself, it's up to you to remember to reposition her. Pad bony areas such as hips, heels, between knees and ankles.

If Alice is able to turn herself, don't let her lie on her favorite side too long. Remind her to turn. If she is unable to comprehend these instructions, prevent her turning after repositioning by the strategic use of pillows. Wedge one or two behind her back to keep her lying on her side.

Her skin should be kept clean and dry - moisture softens skin, making it more easily damaged by rubbing (shearing) or pressure. If Alice is incontinent, there are many products available to help keep her clean and dry. Contact her doctor or home health nurse if you need advice on what to use.

In most cases, decubitus ulcers are a result of neglect. Alice's caregiver may not be turning her often enough. If Alice is incontinent, allowing her to remain wet or soiled, in an effort to save diapers or pads, puts her at risk of developing decubitus. The cost of treating decubitius wounds far exceeds any savings achieved by skimping on diapers or pads.

Other methods of preventing skin breakdown and reducing pressure *(to help treat or prevent decubitus)* include the use of special air or water mattresses, pads and cushions. Find out what is available. Many insurance companies will pay part or all of the cost of these - particularly when it is pointed out that prevention will cost them less in the long run.

Medical attention is needed at the first sign of Stage II or more severe decubitus. Also needed are preventive measures - try to determine what is causing the injury and take steps to change or remove it. Home health nurses, physical therapists and physicians should all be able to offer advice on what to do.

WRITE NOTES HERE

CHAPTER 14

GETTING DRESSED

Styles For Easier Dressing

Most everyone has heard the jokes about hospital gowns that leave your backside exposed. Yes, it's a joke . . . but *is* annoying, embarrasing, and certainly uncomfortable.

Recently, some clever person designed normal looking nightgowns that still open in the back but provide better "covering power". Some fasten with Velcro®, others with snaps or ties. Since they slip on easily from the front, these gowns are ideal for Alice if she can't raise her arms very well. Gowns and robes with long front zippers are also excellent choices.

Even button front pajama tops are a good choice.

When dressing Alice, always remember, "Worst First."

If Alice's arm is paralyzed by a stroke, injury, or stiffened by arthritis, start with it first, when she puts on her gown, robe or pajamas.

The same is true for pullover sweaters and sweatshirts. First slip the sleeve over the affected arm. Then, over Alice's head. Follow with her good arm, then pull it down the rest of the way.

Reverse the process to remove clothing. Get the good arm out first. Then over the head for pullovers. Now pull Alice's affected arm from its sleeve.

If Alice wears bras, look into the styles which fasten in the front. She may be able to put one on by herself. Pullover sports bras offer especially good comfort and support but can be a bit trickier to put on.

Alice can conserve her energy by donning her underwear and pants simultaneously. Start with Alice lying on her back, knees bent. Slip underwear over one foot, then the other. Do the same with Alice's pants, gathering up each leg so it slips on quickly. Pull underwear up as far as possible, followed by the pants. If Alice is able, she now raises her hips. Again, slip underwear up first, then the pants.

If Alice is unable to raise her hips, get both garments over her feet as described above. Pull them up as far as possible. Using the draw sheet (*Chapter 11 : Urinary*

Incontinence, Using a Draw Sheet to Turn Alice) with gentle pressure on Alice's hip and shoulder, turn her on her side. Pull up underwear and pants on the top side. Roll Alice onto her other side and pull both garments up on that side. Several turns back and forth may be required to get both garments comfortably in place. Make sure there are no wrinkles to irritate Alice's skin. Be particularly alert for rolled elastic, such as in waist bands, which can be especially bothersome.

If Alice is able to sit on the side of the bed and stand up, putting on pants is even easier. Before sitting up, Alice should do 5-10 ankle pumps. These are described in the next chapter *(Chapter 15: Getting Out of Bed)*.

Once she is sitting up, slip Alice's underwear and pants over her feet and lower legs. Before Alice stands up, put on her socks and shoes or slippers. Make sure that socks or stockings don't have tight elastic that can constrict circulation. After Alice's footwear is in place, she can stand up - using her walker for support if she has one - while you pull up her underwear and pants. Wearing everyday "normal" clothes will make Alice feel better about herself and promote a positive attitude. Get her dressed even if she is bedridden, unless she has severe pain or is comatose.

Now is a good time to mention the importance of maintaining a routine. Try to get Alice bathed, dressed, and out of bed at the same time every morning. Of course, "same time" does not necessarily mean "early." Try to get her up at

6:00 a.m. and she might smack you with her catheter bag. The point is, don't let her lie around in bed all morning if she is capable of getting up. Maintaining a routine and getting out of bed every day promotes a positive attitude. It also prevents bed sores and weakness.

WRITE NOTES HERE

CHAPTER 15

GETTING OUT OF BED
& THE NEXT "STEP"

Now just look at Alice. She's been brushed, scrubbed, rolled around and dressed. Take a minute to catch your breath.

It's time to get Alice out of bed. Here's how.

HOW TO DO IT – STEP-BY-STEP

GETTING OUT OF BED

If she has a hospital bed raise the head up so Alice is in a sitting position. Lower the foot; no sense in climbing over any mountains. Let Alice adjust to her new position so she doesn't get dizzy.

1. Sit Alice on the side of the bed. Let her do it herself if she can.

She can't? If you are standing at the left side of the bed, grasp Alice's right hand with your right hand, like a handshake. *See Figure T1* This gives you the best leverage. Be careful, though; Alice may have an arm affected by a stroke or other injury. *Don't pull on an affected limb.*

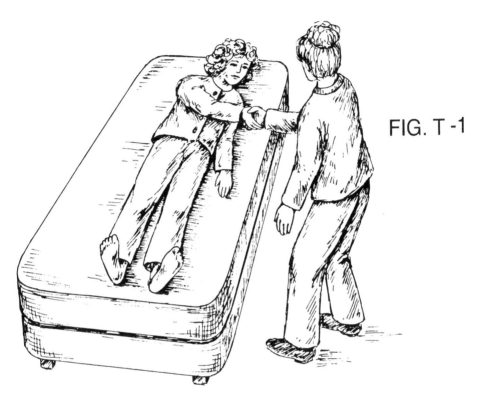

FIG. T-1

2. Pull gently as Alice slides her feet off the bed and pivots toward you. She should attain a sitting position without too much effort. *See Figure T2*

3. Let her take a breather. Be sure her feet are flat on the floor so she doesn't slide out of bed. Use a footstool if Alice's feet don't reach the floor. *Remember to push it out of the way before she stands up.*

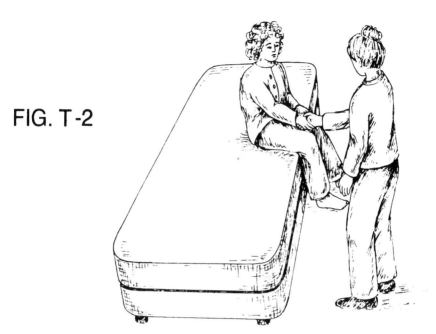

FIG. T-2

4. If Alice stands up too quickly, she may get dizzy and fall down, so let her sit on the edge of the bed for a minute. While she waits she can do ankle pumps to help get her blood circulating and prevent further dizziness.

ANKLE PUMPS

To do ankle pumps, Alice points her toes down as far as she can, then flexes her feet so her toes are pointing up. Repeat 5-10 times. If she is unsteady she can do these even before she sits up. Ankle pumps also limber up ankles and calves. *See Figure U*

Ready to go? Maybe.

85

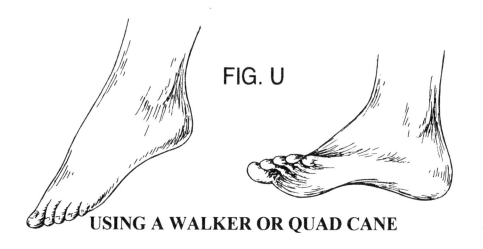

FIG. U

USING A WALKER OR QUAD CANE

If Alice uses a walker we'll hope she's been instructed in it's proper use. This can be done by a home health nurse, physical therapist or a physician. Here's a few reminders.

Alice should not carry the walker. She should set the walker ahead of her and then walk up to it. One foot, then the next. Step. Step. No more than that. Alice shouldn't lean over when she uses the walker. If she does, it is too low or it is too far from her. Periodically check that the walker is bolted together tightly and that all four rubber feet are intact.

If Alice uses a wheeled walker, a little extra attention is required. In most cases, wheeled walkers are not recommended - the risk of their rolling too far from Alice makes them potentially dangerous. However, should Alice be the type who uses a regular walker, but insists on carrying it around instead of using it properly, a wheeled walker might be a good choice for her.

The rules for using wheeled walkers are much the same; Alice moves the walker a short distance, then steps up to it.

If Alice has only one usable hand or arm, a device called a *quad cane* – so called because it has four small feet or legs - might be a better choice than either type of walker. A home health agency or physical therapist can evaluate Alice to see which best suits her needs.

THE NEXT "STEP"

When she is up and about, Alice should wear non-slip shoes. And, absolutely no barefootin' for diabetics or anyone with circulatory problems.

If Alice has a catheter, hook it over the lower cross bar of the walker; it should be placed below bladder level. There should be no tubing hanging down to trip her. Make sure there is no tension on the catheter.

If she uses a cane, somebody will get to carry the catheter bag . . . guess who! The same rules apply when the bag is carried: below bladder level, no tension on the catheter, and keep the tubing from tripping Alice. Now . . . she's off!

But she's kind of wobbly. Maybe Alice doesn't use a walker. Or perhaps she has had a stroke and uses a cane. Is it safe for Alice to walk by herself? Well, you can support her while she walks without destroying your back. Here's how.

Think about the position in which your arms and hands can exert the greatest amount of force. You open jars in front of you, between waist and chest level, not over your head, not at shoulder height and not behind your back. So, your greatest strength is right around chest level, and you should support Alice from this position.

How? First gently bend Alice's affected arm at the elbow. Then cup her elbow in the palm of your hand. A steady pressure upward on her elbow will raise that shoulder so that it is even with her good shoulder. This helps Alice balance.

Suppose Alice's affected side is her left. Cup her left elbow with your left hand. This will position you behind Alice and slightly to her left side. See Figure V

FIG. V

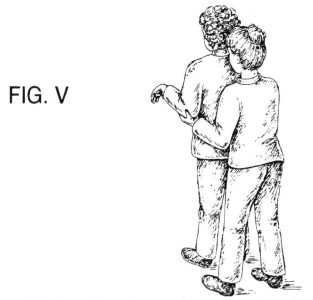

Place your right hand on her waist or back to further steady her. If you really feel she might fall, grip her clothing.

Should Alice start to fall you are prepared. It also means you won't make a grab for her and give her a good pinch while trying to catch her. Better still, use a *gait belt*. These wide sturdy belts are used by physical therapists to help patients maintain their balance. Any secure wide belt that you can hold on to will do the trick. It should be made of a non-stretch material. Canvas luggage straps from an army surplus store are an excellent choice and are easily adjusted.

If she doesn't have an affected side but needs assistance, support Alice on your strongest side. The technique of supporting Alice by the elbow is helpful when traveling through narrow hallways or furniture crowded rooms. Another benefit is less strain on Alice's shoulder than if you were supporting her underneath the affected arm. This also reduces the chance of dislocating her shoulder.

What if Alice starts to fall and you can't seem to stop her? Don't be a hero . . . or an idiot. Don't throw yourself on the floor to cushion her fall unless you have good disability insurance and are ready for a long vacation.

But neither should you abandon Alice and let her bounce on the floor. Keep your grip. Try to get an arm around her. Use the strength of your legs to reduce the speed of her fall, and, as gently as you can, ease her to the floor. Make her comfortable and then call for help. Be prepared, and have emergency numbers at hand before you need them.

CHAPTER 16

WHEELCHAIRS: TRANSFERS & SAFETY

Transfers are exactly what they sound like. You are physically transferring Alice from one place to another. Whether the transfer is from bed to wheelchair, or wheelchair to toilet, or . . . it is important to practice good body mechanics. This means you should use your body the smart way:

- Take advantage of the fact that your legs are stronger than your arms or back.

- Be aware that it is easier to move Alice if you are close to her, rather than at arms' length.

- Always keep your back straight with your knees slightly bent.

- Keep your feet shoulder width apart to provide a broad base of support for strength and balance.

- If you have to lift something heavy, from the floor, squat to reach it, keeping your back vertical; do not bend at the waist. And then slide the object up onto your knee or thigh before standing, to bring it closer to your body.

- When lifting something – or someone – heavy – and you have squatted to pick it up, make sure that your bent knees are pointing in the exact same direction as your feet.

Pivot Transfers

Let's look at transferring Alice from bed to wheelchair. *(It's basically the same as moving her to a regular chair, so we won't cover that separately.)*

PREPARATION

First, get the wheelchair ready. If there is a cushion or covering over the seat, make sure it is in place, with no wrinkles. A piece of a foam egg crate mattress works well for this - it doesn't slide. And it helps keep Alice in the chair. A towel, pillow case, or any other suitable covering can be spread over the top of the foam rubber for added comfort. Meanwhile, Alice can do 5-10 ankle pumps.

Decide which way you want to turn the chair. If Alice has had a stroke and a leg/arm is affected, you want to position the chair on her good side. Otherwise, go toward your strongest side. Bring it in close, but into a position in which it will not be in the way.

On the side nearest the bed, remove the arm and footrest, or swing the footrest back out of the way. It really doesn't take very long and prevents back strain and banged shins.

Alice should slide her hips over close to the edge of the bed before she sits up. This sets her up for a stable sitting position. Once Alice is brought to a sitting position, angle her so that she only has to turn slightly to be in front of the chair when standing. Let Alice rest and get her bearings while you position the wheelchair. *See Figure W* Put the wheelchair as close to the bed as possible. Engage the brakes.

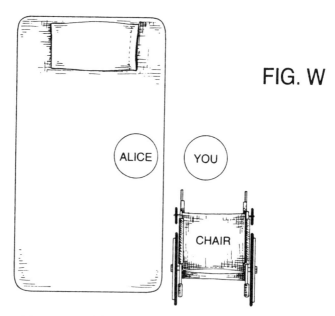

FIG. W

Repeat: Engage the brakes!!!!

OK! Alice is sitting on the side of the bed and wheelchair is in position. She needs only moderate assistance to get into her wheelchair. Here is the best way to give it.

HOW TO DO IT – STEP-BY-STEP

1. Position your foot closest to the chair outside Alice's feet. Your other foot should be between her feet. This keeps feet from getting stepped on and prevents tripping. If you are moving to her left, you should be standing slightly to her left, using your left arm. *See Figure X* for foot position.

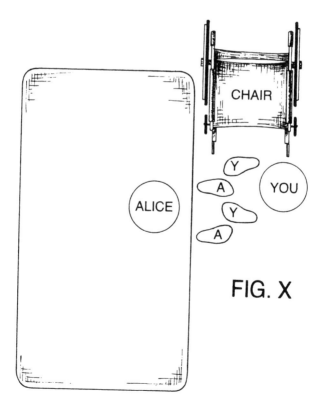

FIG. X

2. Keeping your head up, bend your knees. Keep your back straight. I'll explain more about the importance of this in a moment.

3. Cup her elbow or lift and support her under the arm as she slowly pivots. Do this by hooking the crook of your elbow under her armpit. (*Your* left arm would go under *her* left arm, as you stand toward her left side.)

4. If she is able, Alice can push with her hands on the bed rail, chair arm, or mattress. Or, Alice can balance by holding on to the remaining arm on the wheelchair when it is within easy reach. She should not lean or stretch to reach it.

5. Stand up, using the strength of your legs to help Alice stand. Your knees will still be slightly bent so that you aren't hunched over.

6. Slowly pivot toward the chair until Alice is directly in front of it. Squat slightly (bend those knees) keeping your back straight, and lower Alice slowly into the chair. *No dropping her so she bounces off the seat* (especially since it will be *YOU* who will be the one who has to pick her up off the floor!). She's in. Reattach the armrest and footrest once she is situated.

TWO PERSON TRANSFERS

If Alice is especially large or you are lucky enough to have an extra helper available, "two-man" transfers are the easiest on everyone. Of course, one or both of those "men" can be women.

1. Sit Alice on the side of the bed as in the case of a total transfer. Both lifters should face Alice. The person on Alice's right should slip their right arm (at the elbow) into Alice's underarm. The person on Alice's left should do the same with their left arm. Using some sort of signal, such as counting to three, smoothly lift together and pivot so Alice is in front of her chair.

2. Lower her gently into the chair. The smoother and more coordinated the transfer, the less wear and tear on everyone concerned.

Uh-oh. Alice is sitting crooked. She's too close to the edge. In spite of practice and planning, it happens to the best of us. Transfers can be hard work and don't always turn out as planned.

That's OK. First make sure Alice is not in danger of sliding off. Then put the arm back on the chair. Get behind her. Bend your knees. Reach under Alice's arms and wrap your arms around her chest. The crooks of your elbows should be under her armpits. The crook of the elbow is the strongest lifting point of the arm - it relies on bone strength rather that muscle strength. Keep your head up and neck curved up. Slowly straighten your legs and lift. If she is able, Alice can assist by pushing with her feet and/or hands. *See Figure Y*

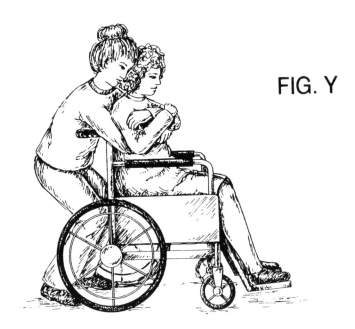

FIG. Y

Oh my! The wheels of the wheelchair seem to have rolled on top of your shoes. Uncomfortable, isn't it? (Alice may not be too pleased either.) What a good way to remember to *ALWAYS* set the brakes before attempting to move anyone into a wheelchair.

Total Transfers

Total transfers are necessary when Alice cannot stand on her own.

PREPARATION

Position the wheelchair and engage the brakes.

HOW TO DO IT – STEP-BY-STEP

1. Alice does 5-10 ankle pumps before sitting up. If Alice can move herself, she should scoot her hips over to the edge of the bed to get into position. A gentle pull from the opposite hand, handshake style, should be enough to bring her to a sitting position. You may have to help her lift her feet out with your other hand - only light support should be needed. As in pivot transfers, angle her so that she won't have to turn a great deal to be in line with the chair. This will save a lot of effort on your part.

2. Get Alice's feet on the floor then give her a second to get her balance.

3. Position your foot closest the chair outside Alice's feet. Your other foot should be between her feet. This is important so you don't trip each other. It also brings you closer to Alice, putting less strain on your back muscles and arms. See Figure X on page 93 for foot positions *(no, we didn't get this diagram from Arthur Murray).*

4. Bend your knees, not your waist or back. Hug Alice around the waist. Keep your upper back straight, your head up, and watch where you are going. Grasp your wrist with your other hand. Alice can hug you around the shoulders - she should be leaning slightly forward. Do not let her hug you around the neck *(it causes you to hunch over and use your back muscles instead of your legs).* See Figure Z

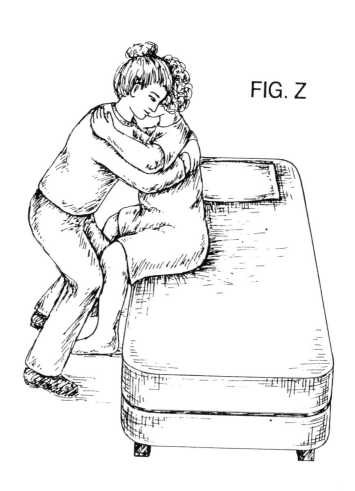

FIG. Z

The importance of keeping your head up when transferring bears repeating. Your neck should actually curve up, causing your spine to form an "S" shape. As explained by a physical therapist, keeping the head up curves the cervical spine (the neck region) causing the vertebrae of the lumbar spine (your lower back – you know, the spot that always aches after you've been lifting heavy stuff) to lock. This means the bones actually support more of the weight, taking strain off the muscles. So remember, heads up!

5. Stand up, taking Alice's weight on your legs. Keep your knees slightly bent to prevent leaning forward. Slowly pivot toward the chair until Alice is directly in front of the chair. Squat slightly, keeping your back straight, to lower Alice into the chair. *She's in.*

6. Attach the foot rests. Make Alice comfortable. Would she like a cushion under her elbows? If she is a stroke patient, prop her affected hand on a cushion or pillow to prevent swelling. Doctors use a two dollar word for this type of swelling - *edema.* Her hand should be slightly higher than her elbow. If Alice wants a blanket over her lap, make sure it doesn't get tangled up in the wheels.

An Alternative Total Transfer

What if Alice doesn't have sufficient leg strength to support herself when on her feet? Here's how to deal with that.

HOW TO DO IT – STEP-BY-STEP

1. **Get ready.** Sit Alice up, if she can balance well enough to safely sit on the side of the bed. Get the wheelchair ready – remove the arm and foot and *engage the brakes.*

2. Position your feet outside of Alice's feet, *her* knees between *your* knees. Bend your knees, keeping your head up. Wrap your arms around Alice, under her arms. If you can reach all the way around her, use your dominant (writing) hand to grasp the wrist of your other hand, making for a no-slip grip.

3. **Stand slowly and smoothly.** As you raise Alice to her feet, grip her knees firmly between yours. This helps Alice's legs from buckling beneath her. It also increases your control over where Alice's feet go. This technique is especially useful in confined areas where only one person can fit to perform a transfer.

4. Pivot Alice toward her chair, using your legs and knees to get her into position.

5. Slowly bend your knees, lowering Alice into the chair. Remember to keep your head up.

6. Put on the finishing touches – reattach the footrests and armrests. Arrange any cushions or small blankets that Alice might like to have.

Wheelchair Safety

Let me start by telling you another true story. Once upon a time (sorry, I just had to start that way) I got a patient all cleaned up and transferred him to his wheelchair. After he was situated in the chair, we went outside *via* the ramp his family had built for him. Since he was a stroke patient, I drove. We started down the ramp, which was pretty steep. Suddenly, my hands held nothing more than the two rubber handgrips from the wheelchair. The chair, without handgrips, but with patient, was rolling quite rapidly down the ramp!

I did catch him before any serious damage was done. But after that adventure, I made it a practice to check the handgrips on wheelchairs. If the handgrips on Alice's chair are loose, get new ones, or clean the old ones and glue them on with a waterproof glue.

Periodically check the wheelchair to make sure there are no sharp edges anywhere that you or Alice could make contact with. Make sure the seat and back are not torn or split. Check the wheels. Are the tires worn? Any spokes broken or bent? Is either of the wheel rims bent or warped? Any of these could be dangerous. And . . . oh yes, it would be nice to be *certain* that the brakes work!

Always remember to remove the footrests when transferring Alice to or from the chair . . . or at least swing them back out of the way. **Remove the armrest (on the side closest to her) before transferring Alice to the chair.** That way, if you drop her during the transfer, Alice won't end up with the arm of the chair up her rear. It happens. And it hurts.

Often, wheelchair arms are reversible, with a high end and a low end. Try both positions, to see which Alice finds most comfortable.

If Alice tends to slide out of the chair, consider using a piece of foam rubber such as you would cut from an egg crate mattress, as we discussed earlier. Another option is a seat belt. This can be a strap from a home health supply store. Or it can be a sheet folded and tied behind the chair. Position it low, where her lap bends, not around her waist. These seat belts also prevent injury if Alice is an Alzheimer's patient and won't stay in her chair. *See Figure AA*

FIG. A A

Restraint devices should be used for Alice's safety, not as a punishment. Restraints are intended for temporary use, to prevent injury, when Alice cannot be closely attended. Do not use them as a substitute baby sitter. If lap restraints are not used properly and checked periodically, Alice can slide down under them and possibly be choked.

WRITE NOTES HERE

CHAPTER 17

THE HOYER LIFT

What if Alice is unable to get out of bed either by herself, or with your assistance? Is she doomed to lay there forever? Nope.

There is a contraption called a Hoyer lift, which will help you get her out of bed. It consists of a metal framework on wheels, and works something like a hydraulic jack. A sling for Alice to sit in is attached to the lift by straps or chains. See Figure BB Once you learn how to position Alice in the sling and attach it to the lift, you've won half the battle.

Hoyer lifts are simple devices to operate. More importantly they work. The Hoyer lift is also useful when Alice's primary care giver is unable to lift Alice and has no one available to help.

For example, I have used Hoyer lifts to move patients weighing over 300 pounds. Earlier I mentioned being 5'1" and around 110 lbs. Or I was when I started writing this - I will avoid commenting on what sitting in front of a computer for months can do for the figure.

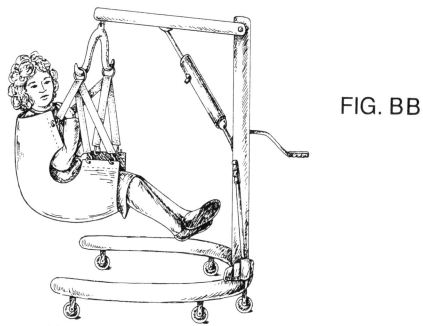

Lifts are also a lifesaver if Alice has had one or both legs amputated. I have had several patients who faced this challenge. The lift made the difference between being in bed 24 hours a day or being able to get around in a wheelchair.

If you feel Alice might be a candidate for a Hoyer Lift, contact her physician, home health agency or a home health supply company. In some cases, Medicare or Alice's private health insurance will pay some of the costs.

Note that there IS a top and bottom to the sling. If the sling has a large opening in one half, that is the bottom. The opening is there to allow Alice to be moved to a bedside commode while in the lift. Naturally, her gown/dress should be pulled up in back or her slacks pulled down first.

If the sling does not have a large opening in one half, it usually has two small holes on each side of the bottom half for attachment of straps/chains. The top usually has three holes. You only use one of the top two holes. Why three? It makes a difference in how upright Alice ends up when she gets lifted.

Here is how to get Alice out of bed using the lift, preferably after she is bathed and dressed.

PREPARATION

Lower the head and foot of the bed, if it is a hospital bed. This makes it easier for her to turn/be turned from side to side.

HOW TO DO IT – STEP-BY-STEP

1. Roll Alice onto her side.

2. Take the sling portion only and roll it in half. Alice likes to have it padded with a soft blanket folded to fit; just roll it all up together, with the blanket next to Alice. *(A blanket is advisable if Alice wears a gown most of the time. If she wears regular clothing the blanket probably isn't necessary.)*

   Keep blanket and sling as wrinkle free as possible. Tuck the rolled portion against her; it should reach from about mid-thigh to about shoulder blade level.

3. Roll her to her other side – over the rolled sling and padding.

4. Move to the other side of the bed and unroll the sling. Again, smooth out blanket and sling. Alice may now lie on her back.

5. Move the lift into position over the bed.

   The bar to which the sling is attached should be centered roughly over Alice's stomach. *Be careful not to smack Alice in the head with the bar!* It is advisable to leave the straps or chains off the bar until after the lift is in place.

6. Lower the bar with the release knob or lever.

7. Now attach the straps. If there are hooks, make sure they point away from Alice once the straps are in place. Attach the shortest strap/chain to the top, the longest to the top hole in the bottom, and the middle length to the last hole in the bottom. If there are only two straps/chains, use the shortest at the top, the longest at the bottom. The idea is to bring Alice into a sitting position.

8. At this point you can use the hospital bed, if Alice is in one, to bring her to a sitting position. This isn't vital, just more comfortable. It is also helpful to lower the hospital bed to its lowest level; that way you won't have to raise Alice so high up in the air.

9. Next, pump the lever to raise the lift bar. Make sure the valve or lever is closed, or the bar will go right back down. Pump until Alice is suspended in a sitting position over the bed. There's no need to pump until she flies up to the ceiling; pump just enough for her behind to clear the mattress.

Be sure Alice changes positions slowly to continue to prevent dizziness. If Alice does become dizzy, she should lean forward and put her head down. Before the transfer, Alice should do ankle pumps to prevent dizziness.

10. Slowly lift her feet off the bed with your hands and pivot Alice until her feet are off the bed. The lift bar will turn with her.

11. Grab the lift by the handles and slowly pull the lift out from under the bed. It pulls easier than it pushes, so have her chair close to the bed. Be sure to allow enough room to maneuver.

It doesn't hurt to practice this part without Alice in the lift. Load something heavy in the sling to make it more realistic Grandkids are often willing guinea pigs. Teenagers are of a good size and weight, though not always as willing, being a breed apart from the rest of the human race.

Remember to make turns slowly. Before you start moving the lift make sure all cords and rugs are out of the way. It is difficult, if not downright impossible, to roll a loaded Hoyer lift over cords or rugs. *The last adventure you want is to flip the lift onto the floor with Alice in it.* If the loaded lift seems kind of tipsy or if Alice is very heavy, and if you have to travel very far, lower her a little and open the legs of the lift *(described in the next paragraph).* A lower center of gravity with a broad base of support is more stable.

12. Position the lift in front of the wheelchair. There is a lever which operates the two legs of the lift. This lever spreads the legs apart, so the lift can be pushed around the chair. The wheelchair can be rolled underneath it, being easier to move than the lift. *Make sure the brakes on the wheelchair are engaged.*

13. Get Alice centered over the chair. You want to position yourself so you can steady Alice with one hand and operate the release lever on the lift with the other. The best place to stand is to one side of the lift.

   Be careful to prevent bumping, pulling or pinching. Be aware of the location of catheter tubes and bags. Avoid the temptation to plop the bag in Alice's lap when loading her into the lift - the urine will re-enter her bladder; result: infection. Instead, hang the drainage bag on the lift itself, at a point lower than Alice's hips.

14. *Reminder: Be sure the brakes on the wheelchair are engaged.* Slowly turn the release knob or push the release

lever, depending on the type of lift you are using. Watch as you slowly lower her into the wheelchair. If Alice looks like she will end up on the edge of her chair, put gentle pressure on her knees to push her well back into the chair. There is no need to push until just before she reaches the chair. You want to get her hips well back into the chair so she won't be slumped over. If she lands too close to the edge, lift her up some and try again.

The raising and lowering steps can be practiced over the bed until both you and Alice are more comfortable with the operation of the lift.

15. Unhook the straps from the bar. For now, hang them over the arms of the chair. Back the lift away from her, again being careful not to smack Alice in the head with the bar. To keep the bar from swinging around, you can secure it to the arm with a piece of string or cord. *(No, not your arm, the arm of the lift!)*

The straps can be removed or left attached to the sling. Reattaching them can sometimes be difficult. If left on, make sure they aren't poking Alice or are at risk of becoming tangled in the wheels of her wheelchair.

Believe it or not, operating a lift can become easy. With practice you can transfer Alice in a matter of minutes. Do remember, that if the phone rings or someone knocks at the door while Alice is in the lift . . . let it ring or let them knock. You don't want to leave Alice unattended while suspended in mid-air. A door intercom and cordless telephone can make life with Alice a lot easier.

If Alice is going to be sitting for any length of time, be sure to position her comfortably in the chair. Her back should be supported. Alice's arms, legs and feet should also have support. Cushions under her arms or elbows can prevent shoulder and neck strain. Propping feet and legs on a stool or foot rest can prevent swelling of feet and ankles. Remember Alice's knees should be slightly bent; a pillow behind her knees helps.

Great! By one means or another, Alice is now in her wheelchair. She's ready to roll, isn't she? Well . . . maybe not. Before we send Alice on her way, be sure to make sure she is safe in her wheelchair *(Chapter 16: Wheelchairs: Transfers & Safety).*

WRITE NOTES HERE

CHAPTER 18

WHEN THEY CAN'T GET OUT OF BED

There are some instances when Alice is completely bedbound, perhaps due to severe pain or weakness resulting from a terminal illness. If Alice cannot get out of bed, it is very important to reposition her every two hours or so. If she is able to move around and turn herself, remind her to do so. Repositioning helps prevent pressure sores, known more commonly as bedsores *(decubitus ulcers). (See Chapter 13: Decubitis Ulcers: Prevention and Treatment)*

These enemies of the disabled can show up on heels, ears, elbows and over the hip bones. In short, just about any part of the body not well padded. Even soft, cushioned areas can be affected.

The primary warning sign of pressure sores is reddened skin. Check these areas when you turn Alice. Gentle massage with lotion or powder will help maintain the circulation, keeping Alice's skin healthy and whole. *Remember, don't rub reddened areas.* If she is incontinent of urine or stool, or if she perspires heavily, Alice is particularly at risk for bedsores.

Another enemy of the bed bound and the inactive homebound is foot drop. Most common in the bed bound, this condition results when muscles in the backs of calves shrink in length due to lack of use. When you go to bed tonight, lie on your back and get comfortable. Then, think about what your feet are doing. Most of us, Alice included, tend to let our ankles relax. Our feet and toes point down. Try it for 24 hours a day, every day and see what happens. They get stiff. Soon the toes stay pointed.

If Alice developed foot drop while recovering from surgery or illness, she might regain her strength only to find out she couldn't stand up. Unless you are a ballerina, you don't walk on your toes. Several steps (no pun intended) can help prevent foot drop from occurring.

FIRST, reposition, reposition, reposition. Alice is less likely to develop toe pointing when she lies on her side.

SECOND, put shoes on her. When she is in her chair Alice can wear shoes . . . who says she can't wear them in bed too? Soft, high top tennis shoes are perfect for keeping Alice's feet in position. If Alice complains that the shoes irritate her toes, cut the toe box out of the shoes! This will provide ventilation and keep her toes from being restricted.

THIRD, but equally important, is exercise. Ankle pumps (described in *Chapter 14: Getting Dressed*) are effective, even if Alice isn't getting up. They restore circulation and ease stiffness. Any kind of movement helps.

An important point to remember is that Alice's toe pointing may not be caused by foot drop. It could actually result from contractures created by years of wearing high heeled shoes. If this is the case, contact Alice's physician, home health nurse or physical therapist for an evaluation and possible solutions.

Also, when she is lying in bed or sitting in a chair, try to keep Alice from crossing her ankles. This habit seems to increase the risk of developing foot drop.

If Alice is a stroke patient or has an illness which puts her at risk of developing foot drop, she may be fitted with plastic splints which hold her feet in the proper position. These are usually ordered by her physician or physical therapist. Another trick is to insert a board between the mattress and the foot board at the end of the bed. Stand pillows up between this board and Alice's feet, to provide an artificial "floor" which will support her feet.

WRITE NOTES HERE

CHAPTER 19

TIPS TO MAKE LIFE EASIER FOR ALICE AND YOU

Rugs

I'm sure you're familiar with throw rugs. Aptly enough, that's exactly what you should do with them. Throw them - *out.* The attractiveness of these decorative little rugs is not worth the pain and debilitation of a broken hip. Those little charmers tangle up walkers, obstruct wheelchairs and are very dangerous. Look for them in every room in the house, including the kitchen *(those little rugs in front of the sink or stove)*, the front hallway *(to wipe mud and snow covered shoes)*, and the bathroom *(in front of the bathtub, to protect the floor from wet feet, or wet feet from the cold floor!)* See also, Bathroom Safety, a little later in this chapter.

Electrical Cords & Wires

Keep an eye out for rugs' accomplices - electrical cords and wires that can also trip Alice. If possible, get on your knees and drop down to floor level to look for anything that might cause Alice to fall.

Slippery Floors & Sidewalks

It's nice to have clean and shiny, freshly waxed floors . . . unless it is Alice who is trying to walk over them. Maybe you should hold off on the wax for awhile. And try to mop floors when Alice will be resting long enough that they will have time to dry. Alice may not be able to see wet areas on the floor, and she will be at risk for a fall.

If you live in Florida or Southern California, chances are that neither you nor Alice will ever see any snow or ice. Live most other places, and winter snow and ice can turn into a real hazard for Alice if she decides to go outside for a breath of fresh air. A cold night can put a thin coating of ice on the ground, or even on your porch or deck, that Alice won't see until it's too late. If Alice wants to go outside for some fresh air – and that's probably a *GREAT* idea for her – just make sure that *you* are the first one out the door, to check the condition of whatever she will be walking on.

Rest Stops

If Alice is able to be up and around, either with or without your assistance, establish "rest stops" throughout the area in which she will be walking. Position a chair at the halfway point between the bed and the bathroom, for example. Locate a stool in the hallway, perhaps in the doorway of an unused room. How about a chair on the landing of the steps?

These rest stops provide Alice a place to stop and catch her breath while moving about the house. While it may not sound like much, the knowledge that she *might* not be able to make it down a long hallway or up a long flight of steps could very easily discourage Alice from trying. When she stops trying, Alice will only get weaker.

Telephones & Monitors

If Alice must be left alone for any length of time, it might be wise to invest in a cordless phone she can keep with her - in an emergency she can use it to call for assistance. Consider getting a programmable phone – which will allow Alice to dial emergency numbers by pressing just one or two buttons.

Or look into getting a monitoring device that calls for help at the push of a button. Remember the little old lady in the commercial who fell and couldn't get up? Those funny little push button necklaces may not be the height of fashion, but they really work. Most can be set up to contact the fire department, ambulance, police or a family member. Shop around for a reputable service company. Often, this service can be billed to Alice's insurance. The service provider should do the billing for Alice. They should also provide a copy for Alice, so she knows what her insurance is paying for.

Smoke & Carbon Monoxide Detectors

Are there enough smoke detectors throughout the house? Are the batteries functional? Can Alice hear them? It sure won☐t help much if she can't. If Alice hears them can she do something about it? Schedule check dates on the calendar.

Look into carbon monoxide detectors if heating or cooking is done with gas, especially during the winter months, when windows are closed. (It seems Alice complains of being cold all the time, anyway). Detectors are available in stores of every type, these days – hardware, gas company, warehouse clubs and . . . .

You may be able to persuade the gas company to send someone out to inspect the gas heating system for leaks. The main symptoms of carbon monoxide poisoning are feeling very sleepy – and getting headaches. If you think Alice has been exposed to carbon monoxide, get her into fresh air, see a doctor, then contact the gas company.

Alzheimer's Disease

Here's a true-to-life example of the type of totally unpredictable incident that can occur as a result of Alzheimer's Disease.

A patient admitted to our agency - an elderly woman with Alzheimer's - cooked rice for dinner. What was the problem? She put the rice - box and all -on the stove's burner and turned it on! Modern medicine has a long way to go before it understands this disease. At present our only option is to keep individuals with Alzheimer's safe. They can't be left alone.

A friend's grandmother was an Alzheimer's patient. She became an escape artist; this frail little old lady could sneak out and travel several miles on foot. Usually half dressed. Sadly, this seems to be a common habit of Alzheimer's patients. Consider installing locks on attic and basement doorways - to keep Alice from falling down the steps. And consider using alarms on exterior doors - which will sound if Alice touches the doorknob as she tries to get outside. Alarms of this kind, which are designed to be simply hung from a doorknob, are available from electronics stores and mail order catalogs, at a cost of under $10.

Alzheimer's sufferers also seem to have unusual strength. This same frail grandma was able to lift the end of her hospital bed several inches off the floor and bounce it like a basketball. This strength puts the Alzheimer's patient (not to mention the caregiver!) at risk of injury. Consider bolting the bed and other heavy objects to the floor, to reduce that risk.

If Alice's mental capacity is diminished, keep her medication locked away in a safe place. This also goes for cleaning supplies. Ditto for sharp objects, such as knives and the like.

Bathroom Safety

If Alice has to have a rug in the bathroom - perhaps on a cold, and slippery bathroom floor, for example - use a rubber backed type to prevent it from slipping underfoot. Or use a suction cup backed bath mat. *(Who says they're just for bathtubs?)* These non-slip mats are also a must for the tub. To prevent mildew from forming on the back, pull them up after use and hang them over the side of the tub. An occasional spray with disinfectant will help prevent mildew. Mildew resistant mats are also available.

Consider adding a rail around the toilet if Alice is able to get up but is somewhat shaky. There are numerous styles that bolt to walls or fasten directly onto the toilet. As mentioned in another chapter, bedside commodes are convenient if Alice is able to get out of bed yet doesn't have the strength to walk to the bathroom. These help take the risk out of nighttime nature calls.

Please make sure the toilet paper dispenser is convenient and well anchored, as must be the roll of toilet paper itself. It is very frustrating to be enthroned and be reaching for the toilet paper, only to have the roll drop to the floor and take off, bouncing across the room like an errant hockey puck, leaving a trail of tissue in its path.

The only thing worse than a runaway roll of toilet paper, is *no* roll of toilet paper. Make sure that there is always an extra roll of toilet paper *within Alice's reach*. The top of the tank is not a bad place, if Alice can reach around behind her without getting up.

Toilet paper is dry, so it can be very irritating when used for particularly messy occasions. The solution: baby wipes. The generics are inexpensive and contain the same ingredients as name brands; they just don't charge for the advertising. These wipes are especially soothing when Alice has hemorrhoids or diarrhea.

Getting Physical - Breathing & Physical Exercise

Whether bed bound or very active, it is important for Alice to perform range of motion *(ROM)* exercises - moving each part of the body through a range of motion *which is normal for Alice.* Don't expect her to be able to put one foot behind her ear, or do splits, unless that is something she was in the habit of doing before she became homebound.

These exercises can be done by Alice independently - or with your assistance. In either case, remember we are not training for the Olympics here, just preventing stiffness and *contractures.* Contractures are caused by the progressive shortening of muscles and the stiffening of joints, until the joints freeze, preventing motion or movement.

Contact Alice's physician or home health agency for a list of exercises suitable for her condition. If she isn't seen by home health care, contact an area home health agency, health department or rehabilitation facility. Any of these should be willing to provide an illustrated list of exercises.

If all else fails, make a trip to the library. Still no luck? Make up your own. The idea is for Alice to move her arms, legs, neck, etc. in ways both natural and comfortable. Raising and lowering her arms, flexing her hands and fingers, and swinging her feet are all ROM exercises.

Equally important is exercising Alice's lungs by doing deep breathing exercises. Deep breathe, in and out, slowly, ten times. Alice can do these exercises 3 to 4 times a day. If Alice becomes short of breath, help her practice pursed lip breathing. When she exhales, she purses her lips as if blowing out a candle. Alice should try to blow as long as possible. This technique slows air flow and gets breathing back under control. Concentrating on the rhythm can help relax Alice, which also helps her breathing. Help Alice remember the rule my track coaches taught me – in through the nose and out through the mouth (through pursed lips).

WRITE NOTES HERE

CHAPTER 20

COPING WITH Y2K

(AND OTHER POTENTIAL DISASTERS –
NATURAL & "MAN-MADE")

WHAT IS Y2K & HOW WILL IT AFFECT ALICE?

In a nutshell, on January 1, 2000, some computers may think it is January 1, 1900. The result: those computers may *shut down,* or they may *do something different* from what they are supposed to do. This problem will likely affect everyone - *that means you and Alice, too.*

Computer people are working to correct this problem, but there are *millions* of computers to be checked and fixed, including those that control *medical equipment, natural gas pipelines,* and *electrical* and *telecommunications transmission lines.* Guess what…because of insufficient time, or the inability to locate the problem, some computers *won't get fixed* before they fail. For many people this will be an *annoyance.* For others it will be a *significant problem.* For Alice it could be *life threatening.* Here's why.

POWER. If it fails, you could have no way to operate any electric or electronic equipment that Alice needs for her care. A four *hour* battery backup won't help Alice if the power is out for four *days.* To prepare, find a store that sells gasoline powered electric generators. *(Honda makes several compact, reliable units, including a one kilowatt model.)* **Buy one of appropriate size and *test it* to make sure it works properly. Take into account the fact that a generator of sufficient capacity to provide electric power to Alice's medical equipment, is likely *not adequate* to keep you all warm, and/or to operate cooking equipment.**

Place the generator *away from your home* - far enough that deadly *carbon monoxide* from the generator cannot be sucked back into your home. Install a <u>*battery powered*</u> *carbon monoxide detector* to be sure. Note that the greater the distance between the generator and your home, the heavier duty the extension cord you will need to avoid power loss.

Buy enough gasoline to power the generator for as long as you may need it. Liquid gasoline is *FLAMMABLE* and gasoline fumes are *EXPLOSIVE*, so store it carefully. *Before you buy <u>any</u> gasoline, check with knowledgeable authorities on the best and safest way to store it, in your particular situation.*

Gasoline is also an *unstable* substance – it tends to break down and become *unusable*. Prevent breakdown by adding *STA-BIL™*, a gasoline stabilizer designed for use by consumers. *If you store the generator with gasoline in its tank, be sure to add stabilizer <u>and</u> to fill the tank to the very top, leaving as little air space as possible, to minimize the accumulation of explosive gasoline fumes.*

<u>*TELECOMMUNICATIONS*</u>. How would you call for medical or home care advice or assistance if your telephone

didn't work? Cellular phone service, e-mail, and access to the world wide web could also be affected. In the event you *did* have telephone service, but *did not* have power, you can communicate using a *non-electronic* telephone – one *without* an a.c. power cord. Buy one for a few dollars - and test it!

HEALTHCARE SERVICES. According to Senator Robert Bennett *(R. Utah)*, chairman of the Senate committee on Y2K preparedness, the healthcare industry is among the *least prepared* for Y2K. Information published in January 1999, in advance of the final report, indicates that more than 90% of private practice physicians are *unaware* of the potential problems with their computers - which deal wiith all aspects of patient care, including *diagnostic testing*. In addition, nearly 65% of U.S. hospitals have *no plans to test* their preparations for Y2K. And, many makers of biomedical devices have yet to advise the FDA *whether their equipment will function properly* after January 1, 2000. As that date draws near, adminstrators of hospitals, nursing homes, hospices, and assisted living facilities may decide to send patients home to avoid potential problems. *This book will help you care for loved ones at home during that time of uncertainty or in the event real problems arise.*

What else should you do to prepare for Y2K and for any other potential disturbances or disasters? Call your local branch of the American Red Cross and ask them to send you a copy of the disaster preparedness brochure, *Y2K: What You Should Know*. Read it . . . and follow its recommendations.

WHEN WILL THIS PROBLEM START?
WHEN WILL IT END?

Power and telecommunications companies are working very hard to find and solve computer problems, to avoid future outages. But what about the problems they simply don't know exist? And what about the fact that in order to determine whether their "fixes" are working, they have to test their systems *long before* January 1, 2000. Outages can result from tests in which problems were discovered. Outages can occur *now* . . . so the time for you to prepare is *now*.

When will it start? Possibly as early as the first quarter of 1999. When will it end? Perhaps not until the second or third quarter of 2000 – or maybe not even until sometime in the year 2001 or 2002!

Wait, don't panic!!! We're <u>not</u> talking about losing electric power or phone service for two years! We're telling you that the *potential* for a *possible* outage – *which always exists* – may *increase significantly* during that period of time.

It is possible <u>you</u> may not encounter an outage. Or that any outage might last only <u>minutes</u> or <u>hours</u>. But <u>some areas</u> may experience extended outages of several days or longer.

So, don't take chances with Alice's well being. Make like a Boy Scout – *Be Prepared!*

CHAPTER 21

MEALTIME

Several simple, common sense rules can help make mealtime more pleasant for Alice. This, in turn, makes it easier for you.

- If her appetite is poor, offer Alice five to six smaller meals rather than three large ones.

- Avoid heavy, greasy foods.

- Take the time to find out Alice's likes and dislikes.

- If Alice is on a bland or puréed diet, don't make comments about how awful the food looks or smells. Even if Alice is non-communicative, you should always assume she can understand what you say and do. These comments can ruin her appetite. At one time I had the rather doubtful pleasure of working in a nursing home. The most vivid memory of my training period is helping feed a blind patient. She was happily eating her pureed food when one of the attendants made a comment about how awful the food looked. The patient stopped and would not eat another bite. Be a positive force in Alice's life. She may not have very many others.

- The fact that Alice is on a special diet for health reasons - perhaps a diabetic diet or low salt diet or perhaps some other diet restriction – doesn't mean that the food *has* to taste awful. Alice can enjoy many of the foods she has always loved. The change comes in their preparation and the quantities allowed.

Diabetic diets are extremely important. New cookbooks with easier recipes and added variety are being published all the time. Low salt diets are keys to controlling high blood pressure and diseases such as congestive heart failure *(CHF)*, the condition in which the heart no longer beats strongly enough to move Alice's blood around her body. The result is fluid build-up in the body tissue, particularly in the extremities - feet, ankles and hands. This fluid build-up, known as *edema*, makes these areas appear swollen. To check for edema place two fingers on the swollen area and press gently. Hold the fingers there for a few seconds. If your fingers leave a lingering impression, it is a sign of edema.

If edema has just developed, contact Alice's doctor or nurse immediately. If she doesn't have a regular doctor, find her one quickly. In the meantime, prop up the swollen limb on pillows to help relieve the edema. While the condition is generally not life-threatening, it can be serious and requires immediate attention.

CHAPTER 22

BOWELS AND KIDNEYS: KEEP THEM MOVING

Lets talk about elimination of bodily wastes.

For comfortable and regular bowel movements, adequate fiber and fluids are essential. Fruits, vegetables and cereals can provide the fiber. Fruit juices provide some fiber, as well as fluid.

Coffee, tea, soft drinks, and other caffeine laden drinks can actually cause the body to lose more fluid than they add, so be sure Alice drinks plenty of water or juice if she is a caffeine drinker. Watch out for chocolate too – it is loaded with *theobromine*, which mimics the physiological action of caffeine.

If Alice is on any type of special diet, such as a diabetic diet, or is on fluid restrictions, be sure to follow the guidelines provided to you. Remember too, that exercise promotes regularity in elimination.

Drinking plenty of fluids will help Alice's kidneys function properly. If she does not drink a lot, acidic drinks such as cranberry juice can help prevent bladder infections; just keep medical diet guidelines in mind. This is particularly important if Alice has a catheter.

If Alice is bed bound, be sure she is turned every two hours or so. This not only helps prevent pressure sores, it guards against kidney stones. Doctors say that lying on her left side provides Alice with the best kidney function. Exercise improves most all bodily functions, and kidney function is no exception.

WRITE NOTES HERE

CHAPTER 23
MEDICATIONS

Like many elderly patients, Alice takes enough medications to keep a pharmacist busy for hours. If she doesn't use one already, consider getting a pill dispenser which shows the date or time she must take her medication. Label the times/days with a permanent marker. The use of a pill dispenser also makes it easier to project when a refill will be needed.

Make out a medication schedule showing each medication, and the date and time it is to be taken. A large calendar works well. Cross off each dose after Alice takes it. When she goes to the doctor, make sure all of Alice's medications go with her. Take the schedule too. Make sure the doctor looks at them. If the doctor prescribes something new, he'll know what she's already taking and be better able to guard against possible drug interactions. Besides, Alice may still be sitting in the waiting room when her next dose is due.

A very special medication rule to remember is that Alice should have no over-the-counter (OTC) medications without the physician's approval. And, Alice should never use an old medication she has stashed in the back of the medicine cabinet. In fact, you should go through Alice's medicine cabinet and throw out all old medications.

Another rule is that Alice may drink no alcoholic beverages when she is taking prescription or OTC medications. Alcohol can act as a synergist, making the medication more potent than it would be without the alcohol. Recently, researchers discovered that combining acetaminophen (the active ingredient in Tylenol® and in certain other OTC pain medications) with alcohol may be linked to liver damage.

Yogurt was mentioned in *Chapter 8: Mouth Care,* as a cure for thrush. Yogurt can also provide relief for other ailments. Many female patients find plain yogurt helps relieve vaginal yeast infections. On the recommendation of a nurse, I have tried it. It works quite well. It is certainly less expensive than the preparations sold in drugstores. Let the yogurt warm up to room temperature rather than use it straight from the fridge (brrr!). Best results are obtained if Alice uses it at bedtime, or remains lying down for several hours. It can be inserted with a syringe or applicator saved from a yeast medication Alice used in the past.

Yogurt can also clear up yeast rashes under arms, breasts and skin folds. Again, allow it to reach room temperature first. Apply after the affected area has been first washed and dried. One or two teaspoons of yogurt will be enough. Apply the yogurt shortly before bedtime and leave it on overnight. It can be washed off with soap and water the next morning.

Yogurt is good to eat, too. Active culture yogurt helps replace the natural bacteria in our bodies to ward off gastrointestinal ills. Before giving Alice yogurt, *make sure she is not currently taking an antibiotic which specifies no dairy products.*

Another important point to remember: have all your prescriptions filled at one pharmacy; and make sure that the pharmacy uses one of the "new" computer programs which automatically "prevents" the filling of a prescription if potentially harmful interaction between the new prescription and any other current prescription can occur. Pharmacists are usually very busy people and recent studies show that, a fairly large portion of the time, they will not realize that an interaction can occur, unless their computer specifically points it out to them. *Drug interactions can be fatal!*

Along the same lines, be sure that all of Alice's drug allergies, both prescription and OTC, are entered into that same computer.

In these days of managed healthcare, it is likely that you will be forced to switch pharmacies several times during the course of Alice's care. Be sure that *all* the information that is in the former pharmacy's computer is transferred to the new pharmacy's computer when the switch is made. This is not too hard when switching within your neighborhood; it is much more difficult to remember and to do - but every bit as important - when switching to a mail order pharmacy.

And finally, be certain to have all this information on hand to take with you if Alice makes an unexpected trip to the hospital; it could save her life.

WRITE NOTES HERE

CHAPTER 24

CARING FOR THE INNNER ALICE

Alice probably has a lot of time on her hands. Explore different hobbies until you find one that holds her interest. Hobbies not only exercise Alice's mind, they can exercise her joints, as well.

There are books on tape available from the library if she was a reader who now has vision problems. Some organizations offer recordings of the Bible in many different languages at no charge.

Contact local churches and schools for possible visitation programs or even to help with the yard/house work. *IMPORTANT - make sure this doesn't offend Alice's sense of privacy.*

In good weather get out of the house. Go for a drive. Wheel Alice around the block in the wheelchair. Sit outside. Adopt a pet.

Adopt a pet? Sure. If Alice is an animal lover, and is not allergic to the chosen animal, a pet can be a devoted companion. Studies show petting the pooch or cuddling the cat can even help lower blood pressure. Make sure the animal is clean and healthy. Most importantly, it must have a mild disposition.

Consider also, who is going to care for the animal – will there be limitations on their time or ability to do the necessary feeding and caretaking? Remember that cats are self-cleaning, dogs are not. Birds can be cheerful, but their cages will be messy. Watching fish can be restful, but who will clean the tanks? None of these comments is meant to do any more than ask you to determine, in advance of acquiring a pet, how it will be cared for. Don't put a strain on Alice, or her caregiver, by getting an animal whose care is too difficult.

Being homebound likely means that Alice does not get outdoors very much, if at all. The lack of sufficient exposure to sunlight could result in another problem for Alice - *Seasonal Affective Disorder* (SAD). Depression, irritability and other symptoms of SAD, will only serve to increase Alice's misery. A likely solution, once SAD has been diagnosed – exposure to lights that simulate the sun's full spectrum. If you've never heard of this ailment, don't just assume it is unimportant; SAD is far more pervasive than you realize. Remember, for Alice to cope with being homebound, she needs to be happy. SAD can make Alice very sad . . . but you may be able to light up her life with the simple addition of full spectrum illumination.

Of all the things that the inner Alice needs, companionship is one of the most important. There are probably not very many people around to give Alice that companionship. But there *IS* a way for Alice to have dozens . . . hundreds . . . even thousands of "companions." No, it's not the characters in the books that Alice will eventually get tired of reading, but *real people* she can converse with every day.

No, you don't have to worry about huge telephone bills or feeding all these people when they come to "visit." These people can all be found on the *Internet*, in "chat rooms" or at websites where Alice can also find out about things that interest or amuse her. To use the internet, you only need to get a computer – or whatever it takes to get onto the internet at the time you read this book (computers may not be necessary for internet access in the near future). Have someone – one of her grandchildren or the next door neighbor's teen-age kid - show her how to use the internet . . . and get out of her way!

Have you ever heard the phrase, "Laughter is the Best Medicine"? It comes from Readers Digest, and it's the title of the page in every issue that includes "doctor jokes and stories." The sentiment is true – laughter *IS* the best medicine. Does Alice have a sense of humor? Maybe she did in the past, but perhaps her physical problems have become so overwhelming that she doesn't find very many things amusing now. Let her search the internet for humor sites, where she can read thousands of jokes and other "funny stuff." According to one source there are more than 565,000 pages of humor on the internet, all of it easily found and read.

Perhaps the most important thing you can give Alice is your love and respect.

Whether Alice is family or someone who has hired you to care for her, she is a human being. Alice may feel lonely or cut off from the world. Take the time to find out what makes her tick, then wind Alice up. Most of all, don't treat Alice like a child - unless she is one.

Last but not least, take a break. You are important too. Countless times, I have seen family members and caregivers try to assume sole care for a patient. They end up exhausted, and as a result, vulnerable to illness and injury, and very irritable. This is not good for Alice or anyone else. Take some time for yourself. Have someone come in for a few hours so you can get out of the house. You are not abandoning anyone; you are simply taking care of your own mental health. How can you be an effective caregiver it you ignore your own needs. Who will take care of *YOU*?

Respite services are often available from local organizations such as AREA 12 or the Council on Aging. Who knows, maybe Alice will be happy to have you out of her hair for a while!

It is important to remember that you are not alone. Home health care agencies are available to provide skilled care. Treatments formerly requiring hospitalization can now be performed at home. Catheter insertion, wound care, IV therapy, tube feedings, and even certain forms of chemotherapy are just a few such treatments that can be provided in the familiar surrounding of Alice's home. And, home health agencies offer health aides or assistants who can provide personal care for Alice while you take a needed break.

Many agencies have also developed a service known as "extended care." Sitters are available when the main caregiver has to be away from Alice for an extended period of time - at work, shopping or for other reasons. Whatever option you choose, research it well. You are putting Alice's health and safety into someone else's hands. Ask for references - and call them. Request a criminal records check through your local police department.

If you have reason to believe anyone has abused Alice, contact the agency they work for. In the unfortunate event a family member abuses or neglects Alice, contact the health department's social services department or adult protective services. If you cannot find one of these agencies in your community contact Alice'c doctor, the hospital, or the police.

Being a caregiver is not a glamorous job. And it certainly isn't an easy one.

The pay stinks . . . in fact, usually there isn't any pay at all.

Society still considers it a second class occupation, "suitable" only for women.

Just remember that you are greatly appreciated. Be proud, knowing you are doing something not everyone can do.

Even more so, be proud because you have made Alice's life better.

She is at home.

Where she belongs.

Index

142

CONSUMER ORDER FORM

This book is available from retail stores and from select associations and organizations throughout the United States. Use this form to order from the publisher only if you cannot find a local source.

Retailers, associations, and fraternal and business organizations - contact us about quantity discounts for resale or premium use.

Instead of tearing out this page, you may prefer to make a copy on any copying machine. Please use one copy of this Order Form, for *each address* to which copies of this book are to be sent.

_____ x $16.95 . . . . _____
No. of Copies

Postage & Handling { *First* Copy · · · · · · · · · · · · · · · · · ___**$1.05**___

{ *Each* Additional Copy @ $0.50 · · · _____

Sales Tax { *ONLY IF* shipping to an address in Pennsylvania, add 7% Sales Tax · · _____

TOTAL ENCLOSED [_____]

Please enclose payment by check or money order in U.S. dollars. Sorry we cannot accept credit cards or C.O.D.'s. Thank you.

Mail To: ABELexpress • P.O. Box 668, Carnegie, PA 15106 U.S.A.
Have a question? Contact us at: 412-279-0672 or 800-542-9001
412-279-5012 FAX • ken@abelexpress.com

✂ —

THIS IS YOUR MAILING LABEL - PLEASE PRINT NEATLY

_____
Name

_____
Street Address or P.O. Box

_____
City   State   Zip

(____) _____
Telephone - Day *(in case we have a question about your order)*